W9-BAG-667

ASSESSING MEDICAL PREPAREDNESS TO RESPOND TO A

TERRORIST NUCLEAR EVENT

WORKSHOP REPORT

Committee on Medical Preparedness for a
Terrorist Nuclear Event

Georges C. Benjamin, Michael McGeary, and
Susan R. McCutchen, *Editors*

Board on Health Sciences Policy

INSTITUTE OF MEDICINE
OF THE NATIONAL ACADEMIES

THE NATIONAL ACADEMIES PRESS
Washington, D.C.
www.nap.edu

THE NATIONAL ACADEMIES PRESS • 500 Fifth Street, N.W. • Washington, DC 20001

NOTICE: The project that is the subject of this report was approved by the Governing Board of the National Research Council, whose members are drawn from the councils of the National Academy of Sciences, the National Academy of Engineering, and the Institute of Medicine.

This study was supported by a contract between the National Academy of Sciences and the U.S. Department of Homeland Security (Contract HSHQDC-08-C-00014). Any opinions, findings, conclusions, or recommendations expressed in this publication are those of the author(s) and do not necessarily reflect the view of the organizations or agencies that provided support for this project.

International Standard Book Number-13: 978-0-309-13088-2
International Standard Book Number-10: 0-309-13088-3

Additional copies of this report are available from the National Academies Press, 500 Fifth Street, N.W., Lockbox 285, Washington, DC 20055; (800) 624-6242 or (202) 334-3313 (in the Washington metropolitan area); Internet, http://www.nap.edu.

For more information about the Institute of Medicine, visit the IOM home page at: **www.iom.edu.**

The serpent has been a symbol of long life, healing, and knowledge among almost all cultures and religions since the beginning of recorded history. The serpent adopted as a logotype by the Institute of Medicine is a relief carving from ancient Greece, now held by the Staatliche Museen in Berlin.

COVER: The cover depicts a schematic model of the effects of detonating a 10-kiloton (kt) nuclear device at ground level in the central business district of a large metropolitan area. The circles around ground zero represent areas of extensive immediate damage from the blast (red), thermal (orange), and radiation (yellow) effects of the detonation. For illustrative purposes, the circles are not drawn to scale (in a 10-kt detonation, they would be nearly overlapping). The long elliptical contour lines emanating from ground zero represent the area where radioactive fallout would settle soon after a detonation, after being carried by atmospheric winds. The red ellipse represents the area in which the short exposure of anyone outdoors immediately after the detonation would probably be lethal. The orange and yellow ellipses represent areas of progressively less radiation. The H's are hospitals and represent the likelihood that some hospitals, which tend to concentrate in the downtown of most central cities, would likely be affected negatively by a 10-kt nuclear detonation—some by the immediate effects, others by the fallout, and some by both.

Suggested citation: IOM (Institute of Medicine). 2009. *Assessing medical preparedness to respond to a terrorist nuclear event: Workshop report*. Washington, DC: The National Academies Press.

"Knowing is not enough; we must apply.
Willing is not enough; we must do."
—Goethe

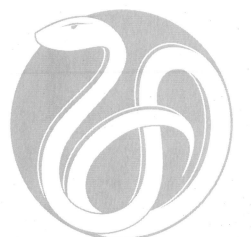

INSTITUTE OF MEDICINE
OF THE NATIONAL ACADEMIES

Advising the Nation. Improving Health.

THE NATIONAL ACADEMIES
Advisers to the Nation on Science, Engineering, and Medicine

The **National Academy of Sciences** is a private, nonprofit, self-perpetuating society of distinguished scholars engaged in scientific and engineering research, dedicated to the furtherance of science and technology and to their use for the general welfare. Upon the authority of the charter granted to it by the Congress in 1863, the Academy has a mandate that requires it to advise the federal government on scientific and technical matters. Dr. Ralph J. Cicerone is president of the National Academy of Sciences.

The **National Academy of Engineering** was established in 1964, under the charter of the National Academy of Sciences, as a parallel organization of outstanding engineers. It is autonomous in its administration and in the selection of its members, sharing with the National Academy of Sciences the responsibility for advising the federal government. The National Academy of Engineering also sponsors engineering programs aimed at meeting national needs, encourages education and research, and recognizes the superior achievements of engineers. Dr. Charles M. Vest is president of the National Academy of Engineering.

The **Institute of Medicine** was established in 1970 by the National Academy of Sciences to secure the services of eminent members of appropriate professions in the examination of policy matters pertaining to the health of the public. The Institute acts under the responsibility given to the National Academy of Sciences by its congressional charter to be an adviser to the federal government and, upon its own initiative, to identify issues of medical care, research, and education. Dr. Harvey V. Fineberg is president of the Institute of Medicine.

The **National Research Council** was organized by the National Academy of Sciences in 1916 to associate the broad community of science and technology with the Academy's purposes of furthering knowledge and advising the federal government. Functioning in accordance with general policies determined by the Academy, the Council has become the principal operating agency of both the National Academy of Sciences and the National Academy of Engineering in providing services to the government, the public, and the scientific and engineering communities. The Council is administered jointly by both Academies and the Institute of Medicine. Dr. Ralph J. Cicerone and Dr. Charles M. Vest are chair and vice chair, respectively, of the National Research Council.

www.national-academies.org

Reviewers

This report has been reviewed in draft form by individuals chosen for their diverse perspectives and technical expertise, in accordance with procedures approved by the National Research Council's Report Review Committee. The purpose of this independent review is to provide candid and critical comments that will assist the institution in making its published report as sound as possible and to ensure that the report meets institutional standards for objectivity, evidence, and responsiveness to the study charge. The review comments and draft manuscript remain confidential to protect the integrity of the deliberative process. We wish to thank the following individuals for their review of this report:

Herbert L. Abrams, Department of Radiology, Professor Emeritus, Stanford University

Brooke Buddemeier, Global Security Directorate, Lawrence Livermore National Laboratory

Michael L. Freeman, Vanderbilt University School of Medicine

Dan Hanfling, Emergency Management and Disaster Medicine, Inova Health System

Nathaniel Hupert, Weill Cornell Medical College

Although the reviewers listed above have provided many constructive comments and suggestions, they did not see the final draft of the report before its release. The review of this report was overseen by **Ms. Hellen Gelband,** Resources for the Future. Appointed by the Institute of Medicine, she was responsible for making certain that an independent examination of this report was carried out in accordance with institutional procedures and that all review comments were carefully considered. Responsibility for the final content of this report rests entirely with the authoring committee and the institution.

Preface

The 20th century brought us the birth of the atomic age, with Albert Einstein's understanding that $E = MC^2$ in 1905, Ernest Rutherford's theory of the structure of the atom in 1911, and the first sustained nuclear reaction in Chicago in 1942. While it brought the promise of a robust use of nuclear technologies for peaceful purposes, it also brought the reality of nuclear weapons in 1945. Those initial weapons were large, heavy, and complex to make and use. Moreover, only nations had nuclear weapons, not individuals or groups. Since then, nuclear weapons technology has continued to advance, producing smaller, lighter, and more potent weapons. In addition to that technological advance, terrorists are working diligently to obtain those devices. Today, the development and detonation of a compact and portable nuclear device by a small group of terrorists is a potential threat.[1] Such an improvised nuclear device (IND) could be small enough to transport in a vehicle and could produce an explosion equal in yield to 10 kilotons (kt) of TNT (trinitrotoluene).[2]

Like other nuclear weapons, an IND detonation would result in substantial structural and environmental destruction from blast, heat, and radiation effects. That destruction would impose a significant additional burden on the normal disaster emergency medical response because of the extent of physical destruction, the presence of dangerous levels of radiation, and the potential loss of critical medical infrastructure in surrounding areas. Numerous operational and logistical problems with delivering supplies, transporting patients, and emergency communications would further complicate the response.

The medical impacts of those injuries are likely to be catastrophic, both for people in the immediate area and for those in a radius of up to several miles. Survivability is related to a combination of the degree and type of injury and the degree of exposure to radiation in both the short and intermediate terms. Those effects have both medium- and long-term health consequences for victims and emergency response personnel. Under any scenario envisioned from the release of an IND, we will have a significant medical disaster with thousands of casualties. The immediate requirement for a large number of specialized beds for burns, broken limbs, head injuries, crushed lungs, eye injuries, and other types of trauma will overwhelm the current health system, which is already overtaxed.[3] The number and variety of casualties, the lack of adequate emergent health care infrastructure in many areas (including burn and trauma beds, respirators, supplies, and trained staff), and the long-term disruption to routine emergent and urgent health care services represent a significant planning challenge.

In addition to the devastation around ground zero from blast, thermal, and prompt radiation effects, a ground-level detonation would create a substantial amount of fallout that would be deposited for miles downwind. Radiation from the fallout would cause death and injury to people exposed to it, especially those outdoors in the first 10-15 miles downwind during the first few hours, but efforts to prepare the public to take the appropriate steps to protect themselves from fallout are almost nonexistent.

Disasters also have serious psychological impacts on people who are involved in them.[4] In general, we are not well prepared to help victims cope with the psychological effects of disasters, and terrorist nuclear events are no exception.

The United States has been struggling for some time to address and plan for the threat of nuclear terrorism and other weapons of mass destruction (WMDs) that terrorists might obtain and use. One of the earliest medical preparedness efforts, the Metropolitan Medical Response System Program, was started in 1995, but it has remained underfunded and its potential has been largely unfulfilled.[5] A range of public health efforts have been taken to prepare for the appearance of pandemic influenza, smallpox, anthrax, and other infectious disease threats. Those efforts have put some systems and some resources in place, such as the National Disaster Medical System, to respond to infectious and other health emergencies, but as Hurricane Katrina showed, they are not adequate to overcome a substantial loss of critical medical and response infrastructure.

There are, of course, a number of public and nonpublic efforts by a variety of federal, state, and local agencies to prevent, mitigate, and respond to the threat of an IND. The latest effort, the Urban Area Security Initiative (UASI), is providing funds to 45 urban areas to improve preparedness for WMDs, including an IND detonation. The Department of Homeland

Security, as directed by Congress, asked the Institute of Medicine (IOM) to conduct a workshop to better understand the state of preparedness for an IND detonation in the six UASI cities designated as "Tier 1." Public health practitioners are usually asked to figure out how to prevent bad things from happening and to preserve our health. The basic assumption for this workshop, however, was to assume: What if? Specifically, what if the efforts by law enforcement and other security officials failed to prevent the detonation of a 10-kt nuclear device in a central city? The committee's task was basically to ask: Where are we today, and what are the gaps should the unthinkable happen? The committee fulfilled that task.

This report provides a frightening but candid look into our level of preparedness today. It was an informative process; one that did much to confirm that we are not yet prepared for a nuclear event. In fact, in many ways, we are still in the infancy of our planning and response efforts. The workshop identified several key areas in which we might begin to focus our national efforts in a way that will improve the overall level of preparedness.

The workshop committee members were a group of some of the most intelligent and wisest people in the areas of emergency preparedness and nuclear response. In addition, the many panel members who contributed to the workshop brought a great deal of technical knowledge and practical reality to the discussion. That contribution was of particular value concerning the status of preparedness of the Tier 1 UASI cities.

In closing, I would like to thank the IOM staff who supported this committee's work, and the committee members with whom I had the pleasure to work. The workshops were complicated, the deadlines tight, and the material complex. The staff did a terrific job, and I was honored to have the opportunity to work with them.

Georges C. Benjamin, M.D., *Chair*
Committee on Medical Preparedness for
a Terrorist Nuclear Event

Endnotes

1. Allison, G. 2004. *Nuclear terrorism: The ultimate preventable catastrophe.* New York: Times Books, Henry Holt and Company; Commission on the Prevention of Weapons of Mass Destruction Proliferation and Terrorism. 2008. *World at risk: The report of the Commission on the Prevention of WMD Proliferation and Terrorism.* New York: Vintage Books; Statement for the Record of Charles E. Allen, Under Secretary for Intelligence and Analysis, U.S. Department of Homeland Security, Before the Senate Committee on Homeland Security and Governmental Affairs, Hearing on *Nuclear terrorism: Assessing the threat to the homeland,* April 2, 2008.

2. Bunn, M. 2008. The risk of nuclear terrorism—and next steps to reduce the danger. Prepared testimony for the Senate Committee on Homeland Security and Governmental Affairs, Hearing on *Nuclear terrorism: Assessing the threat to the homeland,* April 2, 2008.

3. IOM (Institute of Medicine). 2007. *Hospital-based emergency care: At the breaking point.* Washington, DC: The National Academies Press.

4. IOM. 2003. *Preparing for the psychological consequences of terrorism: A public health strategy.* Washington, DC: The National Academies Press.

5. IOM. 2002. *Preparing for terrorism: Tools for evaluating the Metropolitan Medical Response System Program.* Washington, DC: The National Academies Press.

Contents

Tables, Figures, and Boxes

Abbreviations and Acronyms

AFRRI	Armed Forces Radiobiology Research Institute
AMS	Aerial Measuring System
ARAC	Atmospheric Release Advisory Capability
ARS	acute radiation syndrome
ASPR	Assistant Secretary for Preparedness and Response (HHS)
CBRN	chemical, biological, radiological, or nuclear
CBRNE	chemical, biological, radiological, nuclear, or explosive
CDC	Centers for Disease Control and Prevention
CERFP	CBRNE Enhanced Response Force Package
cGy	centigray
CIMS	citywide incident management system (New York City)
CMOC	catastrophic medical operations center (Texas)
CMRT	Consequence Management Response Team
CONOPS	concept of operations
CRAF	Civil Reserve Air Fleet
CRCPD	Conference of Radiation Control Program Directors
CRI	Cities Readiness Initiative
CST	Civil Support Team
DC	District of Columbia
DHS	Department of Homeland Security
DMAT	Disaster Medical Assistance Team (NDMS)
DoD	Department of Defense
DOE	Department of Energy

DRC   Disaster Resource Center
DTPA   diethylenetriamine pentaacetic acid

ED   emergency department
EMAC   Emergency Management Assistance Compact
EMEDS   Expeditionary Medical Support
EMP   electromagnetic pulse
EMS   emergency medical services
EMT   emergency medical technician
EPA   Environmental Protection Agency
ESAR-VHP   Emergency System for Advance Registration of Volunteer
             Health Professionals
ESF-6   Emergency Support Function #6 (NRF)
ESF-8   Emergency Support Function #8 (NRF)
EUA   Emergency Use Authorization

FCC   federal coordinating center (NDMS)
FDA   Food and Drug Administration
FEMA   Federal Emergency Management Agency
FRMAC   Federal Radiological Monitoring and Assessment Center
FY   fiscal year

GPS   global positioning system
Gy   gray

hazmat   hazardous materials
HHS   Department of Health and Human Services
HPP   Hospital Preparedness Program
HSI   Homeland Security Institute

ICU   intensive care unit
IND   improvised nuclear device
IOM   Institute of Medicine
IRB   institutional review board

JumpSTART   Simple Triage and Rapid Treatment (pediatric)

KI   potassium iodide
kt   kiloton(s)

LACDPH   Los Angeles County Department of Public Health

mGy   milligray

MMRS	Metropolitan Medical Response System
mph	miles per hour
MRC	Medical Reserve Corps
mSv	millisievert

NDMS	National Disaster Medical System
NIH	National Institutes of Health
NRAT	Nuclear/Radiological Advisory Team
NRC	Nuclear Regulatory Commission
NRF	National Response Framework
NVHA	Northern Virginia Hospital Alliance
NYCDOH	New York City Department of Health and Mental Hygiene
NYSDOH	New York State Department of Health

OSHA	Occupational Safety and Health Administration

PAG	protective action guide
PAG Manual	*Manual of Protective Action Guides and Protective Actions for Nuclear Events* (EPA, 1992)
PF	protection factor
PHEP	Public Health Emergency Preparedness
P.L.	Public Law
PPE	personal protective equipment
psi	pounds per square inch
PTSD	posttraumatic stress disorder

QF	quality factor

R&D	research and development
rad	radiation absorbed dose
RAP	Radiological Assistance Program
RDD	radiological dispersal device
RDF	rapid deployment force
REAC/TS	Radiation Emergency Assistance Center/Training Site
rem	roentgen equivalent man
REMM	Radiation Event Medical Management
RHCC	regional healthcare coordinating center (Northern Virginia)
RITN	Radiation Injury Treatment Network
RSS	receipt, stage, and storage (site) (SNS)
RTR	Radiation Treatment, Triage, and Transport (system)

SFDPH	San Francisco Department of Public Health

SI	Système International d'Unités (International System of Units)
SNS	Strategic National Stockpile
SRT	Search Response Team
START	Simple Triage and Rapid Treatment (adult)
Sv	sievert
TOPOFF	Top Officials
UASI	Urban Area Security Initiative
U.S.	United States
USPS	United States Postal Service
VA	Department of Veterans Affairs
WMD	weapon of mass destruction
WMD-CST	Weapons of Mass Destruction Civil Support Team

Assessing Medical Preparedness to Respond to a Terrorist Nuclear Event: Workshop Report

INTRODUCTION

A nuclear attack on a large U.S. city by terrorists—even with a low-yield improvised nuclear device (IND) of 10 kilotons (kt) or less—would cause a large number of deaths and severe injuries. A major source of these acute casualties would be the immediate effects of an IND detonation caused by blast overpressure and winds, thermal radiation, and prompt nuclear radiation. Another source of casualties—if the IND was detonated at or near ground level—would be the fallout (i.e., radioactive particles) that would be deposited on the ground for many miles downwind of the detonation point. The heaviest and therefore most dangerous particles of fallout would be on the ground for nearly 10 miles downwind within minutes. The number of casualties from this secondary source could also be of great magnitude. However, the count could be reduced substantially if individuals swiftly took appropriate steps to protect themselves.

Of greatest concern is that, beyond all of the immediate deaths, the large number of injured from an IND detonation would be overwhelming for local emergency response and health care systems to rescue, evacuate, and treat, even assuming that these systems and their personnel were not themselves incapacitated by the initial impact of the explosion. Yet to survive in the long term, many people would need immediate treatment, particularly for severe burns and traumatic injuries. In addition, many of the initial survivors would receive high doses of radiation from the detonation or the subsequent fallout. They should be identified rapidly and directed to facilities for the intensive supportive care that they would need to achieve long-term survival when they eventually became ill with acute radiation syndrome (ARS) during the following days and weeks.

Terrorist groups have indicated an interest in using weapons of mass destruction (WMDs), including nuclear weapons, against the United States, although there is no evidence to date to confirm that any particular group possesses nuclear weapons. Considering the inherent difficulties, it is not known whether such a group actually could develop the capacity to carry out such an attack in the near future, and there is a range of views among experts on the extent of the threat (Levi, 2007; Commission on the Prevention of Weapons of Mass Destruction Proliferation and Terrorism, 2008). Gaining access to sufficient quantities of weapons-grade nuclear material is the highest hurdle facing would-be nuclear terrorists, and numerous other hurdles would have to be overcome before a weapon devised from such material could be used. For example, terrorist groups would require the capacity to manufacture a device that would detonate when (and only when) they wanted. They also would have to transport the device into or within the United States and move it to the targeted location without being detected.

The United States has made preventing such an attack a high priority and has a number of programs in place to (1) deny terrorists access to nuclear materials, (2) deter other nations from helping terrorists mount a nuclear attack, and (3) intercept any attack before it can succeed. Still, since no individual preventive measure or even a set of such measures is fail-proof, the question remains: What if prevention efforts fail?

Over the past several years, the U.S. government has made increased efforts to address this question. In 2004-2005, the Department of Homeland Security (DHS) drafted 15 scenarios to be used in conjunction with planning responses to catastrophic events under the National Response Framework (NRF). The scenarios were chosen to "highlight a plausible range of major events such as terrorist attacks, major disasters, and other emergencies, that pose the greatest risk to the Nation."[1] Relevant to the current discussion, Scenario 1 involves the detonation of a 10-kt IND in the central business district of a large city. The NRF also has a Nuclear/Radiological Incident Annex describing the "policies, situations, concepts of operations, and responsibilities of the Federal departments and agencies governing the

---

[1] Strengthening National Preparedness: Capabilities-Based Planning. A DHS fact sheet at http://www.ojp.usdoj.gov/odp/docs/CBP_041305.pdf (accessed June 23, 2009). The planning scenarios themselves are for official use only; thus, the content of Scenario 1 was not referred to in the workshop, although Brooke Buddemeier's presentation contained details on the health effects of the 10-kt detonation in Scenario 1 that are publicly available.

immediate response and short-term recovery activities for incidents involving release of radioactive materials," including IND attacks.[2]

Congressional committees on homeland security have begun to put more emphasis on the nation's capacity to respond to a nuclear event if prevention fails. The conference report on Public Law (P.L.) 110-28 of 2007 directed DHS to model the effects of 0.1-kt, 1.0-kt, and 10-kt nuclear detonations in each Tier 1 Urban Area Security Initiative (UASI) city; assess current response and recovery plans; identify ways to improve health outcomes; evaluate medical countermeasure distribution systems; and develop information strategies for the dissemination of protective actions that the public, medical community, and first responders should take to prepare for and respond to a nuclear event.[3]

The UASI program of DHS currently provides funds to 45 urban areas for equipment, training, planning, and exercises to respond to the impact of WMDs, including (but not limited to) INDs. The six Tier 1 UASI areas are New York City/Northern New Jersey,[4] National Capital Region, Los Angeles/Long Beach, San Francisco Bay Area, Houston, and Chicago.

The same legislation also directed DHS to have the National Academy of Sciences assess the current level of medical readiness to respond to a nuclear detonation in Tier 1 UASI cities. In response to the congressional mandate, DHS contracted with the Institute of Medicine (IOM) of the National Academies to

- establish a committee of experts in emergency medical response and treatment, medical and public health preparedness, health sciences research, and nuclear medicine;

---

[2] The Nuclear/Radiological Incident Annex is at http://www.fema.gov/pdf/emergency/nrf/ nrp_nuclearradiologicalincidentannex.pdf (accessed June 23, 2009). The annex was issued in 2004 and updated in 2008. It assigns federal agency responsibilities in the event of a release of radiation. DHS would be the lead, or "coordinating agency," in responding to a deliberate attack, such as a terrorist IND, and would be supported by other agencies. In other situations the coordinating agency might be the Department of Energy, the Department of Defense, the Nuclear Regulatory Commission, the National Aeronautics and Space Administration, the Environmental Protection Agency, or the Coast Guard, depending on ownership, custody, origin, or location of the radioactive materials in question. Under another NRF annex (Emergency Support Function #8, "Public Health and Medical Services"), the Department of Health and Human Services would lead the public health and medical response, with the support of other agencies with medical assets, in an IND response. See Topic 6, "Federal and State Medical Resources for Responding to an IND Event," for a summary of HHS's plans and assets for an IND event.

[3] The conference report is at http://frwebgate.access.gpo.gov/cgi-bin/getdoc.cgi?dbname=110_ cong_public_laws&docid=f:publ028.110.pdf (accessed June 23, 2009).

[4] After the workshop, the New York City/Northern New Jersey area was split in two, to form seven Tier 1 UASI areas. The Northern New Jersey area was renamed Jersey City/Newark.

- conduct a workshop planned by the committee on medical preparedness for a nuclear detonation of up to 10 kt; and
- prepare a report on the workshop presentations and discussions.

Specifically, DHS asked for the workshop and workshop report to

1. review and summarize the overall emergency response activities and available health care capacity (including shelter, evacuation, decontamination, and medical infrastructure interdependencies) to treat the affected population;
2. examine the capacity and identify gaps in the capability of the federal, state, and local authorities to deliver available medical countermeasures in a timely enough way to be effective;
3. review and summarize available treatments for pertinent radiation illnesses, including the efficacy of medical countermeasures; and
4. appraise the expected benefit of medical countermeasures, including those currently under development.

COMMITTEE PROCESS

IOM and DHS agreed that the workshop would be based on publicly available information. Classified information and sensitive information marked "For Official Use Only" was not presented or discussed at the workshop or used in this report.

Because official estimates of the likelihood of a successful attack on the United States by terrorists using an IND are not public information, this question was not addressed at the workshop. The scope of the workshop was limited to medical public health preparedness *if* such an event were to occur. Thus, the workshop did not address the priority that emergency preparedness planners should give to responding to the threat of an IND or how resources should be allocated among different threats.

IOM formed a committee with the appropriate expertise and experience to plan and conduct the workshop. The committee held a planning meeting in April 2008. The workshop was held in two parts, June and August 2008. The agendas of the two workshop sessions are found in Appendix A, the list of attendees of the workshop sessions in Appendix B, short biographies of speakers and panelists at the workshop in Appendix C, and short biographies of the committee members, consultant, and staff in Appendix D.

The role of the committee was to plan the workshop by deciding on the workshop topics, identifying experts on those topics to speak, developing questions for the speakers to address, and authoring a report of the workshop discussions. Committee members also moderated the presentations and the question-and-answer period that followed each speaker or set of speakers on a specific topic.

This publication is a report provided by the committee to document the workshop discussions. It is not a consensus document expressing committee findings or recommendations. Rather, it summarizes the views expressed by the workshop participants and committee members in their individual capacities. Although the committee is responsible for the overall quality and accuracy of the report as a record of what transpired at the workshop, the views stated in the workshop report are not necessarily those of the committee or IOM.

WORKSHOP ASSUMPTIONS AND TOPICS

After a day's discussion at the planning meeting, the committee adopted certain assumptions to make the scope of the workshop more manageable. These assumptions in turn helped shape the topics addressed in the workshop.

Assumptions

The assumptions adopted for the purpose of workshop discussions were as follows:

1. The yield of the IND that workshop participants needed to address would be equivalent to 10 kt of TNT (trinitrotoluene). This is somewhat less than the 16- and 21-kt yields of the Hiroshima and Nagasaki bombs, respectively.[5] However, it corresponds to the highest yield that Congress directed DHS to use in modeling the effects of nuclear attacks on the Tier 1 UASI cities in P.L. 110-28, and it is also the same as the yield used in the IND planning scenario under the NRF.

2. The attack would be a surprise, with the intent of maximizing the number of casualties and minimizing the chance that the bomb would be found and disarmed before it could be set off and the bombers would be caught.

3. The terrorists would detonate the IND in the central business district or in another densely populated area to maximize the number of casualties.

4. The attack would occur during a workday to maximize the number of casualties, although the terrorist could choose the middle of the

---

[5] The yields were most recently estimated as being between 14 and 18 kt at Hiroshima and between 19 and 23 kt at Nagasaki, each at a 99 percent confidence limit (RERF, 2002:51-52).

night instead, to exploit vulnerability and minimize the chances of interception and capture.

5. The IND would be detonated at or near ground level. This differs from the bombings of Hiroshima and Nagasaki, where the bombs were detonated at altitudes of approximately 1,970 and 1,652 feet, respectively (RERF, 2002:48, 51). Compared with an airburst, the blast, thermal radiation, and prompt nuclear radiation impacts of a ground-level detonation would affect a smaller area, but radioactive fallout (which was negligible at Hiroshima and minimal at Nagasaki) would be considerable and would affect a very large area (Glasstone, 1962:633-634).

6. The workshop would focus on the acute *medical* effects of the explosion and the resulting fallout. These would include blast injuries, burns, ARS, and combinations of these effects. Although decontamination requirements and the long-term effects of radiation exposure on health, particularly cancer, are also matters of serious medical concern, they were not a focus of this workshop.

7. The workshop would also address preparedness to reduce the psychological and mental health impacts of a nuclear event (which are anticipated to be substantial) and to minimize long-term effects.

8. Although the scope of the workshop would be *national* preparedness, it was recognized and assumed that the initial response would be largely *local* and *regional* and that it could take as long as a week before substantial state and federal resources could arrive. This assumption was based on the realization that no city or metropolitan area would be able to respond to a nuclear event alone and that the preparations for such an event would also have to depend on state and federal government involvement and support.

Topics

To respond to the statement of tasks provided by DHS and guided by the assumptions listed above, the committee selected the topics to be addressed at the workshop, which were reflected in the agenda (Appendix A). The topics were the following:

1. Effects of a 10-kt IND detonation on
   a. human health and
   b. the regional health care system
2. State-of-the-art medical care for two mostly distinct groups, namely victims of
   a. the immediate effects of a nuclear detonation (i.e., injuries from blast, heat, and prompt radiation, singly and in combination) and

b.   radiation from the fallout caused by a ground burst
3.   Expected benefit of radiation countermeasures
4.   Potential protective actions and interventions to reduce radiation injury to
     a.   first responders and
     b.   the population under the fallout plume
5.   Risk communication, public reactions, and psychological consequences of an IND event
6.   Federal and state medical resources for responding to an IND event
7.   Current preparedness for responding to the medical needs of those injured by the *immediate* effects of an IND detonation, including the capacity
     a.   to reach, triage, and stabilize those injured by the detonation safely;
     b.   to evacuate casualties to regional treatment facilities;
     c.   of the metropolitan region's medical system to treat casualties; and
     d.   to evacuate serious casualties to appropriate treatment facilities statewide and nationally
8.   Current preparedness to prevent and treat *delayed* casualties caused by radioactive fallout as well as the psychological effects of an IND event

TOPIC 1: EFFECTS OF A 10-kt IND DETONATION ON HUMAN HEALTH AND THE AREA HEALTH CARE SYSTEM

The June workshop began when Daniel Flynn, the committee member who moderated this session, briefly summarized the health effects of an IND detonation. With an IND detonation, he noted, there would be an overwhelming number of casualties with physical trauma and thermal burns with radiation injury, and severely damaged infrastructure. Initially, the preplanned medical response would not be able to match the medical needs. In that vacuum, spontaneous individual responses would be likely from local medically trained and untrained personnel who would step forward to augment the initial emergency medical response (this was seen, for example, at Hiroshima).

Even with volunteers, in an overwhelming mass casualty scenario there would be austere medical care rather than ideal standard-of-care practice. Flynn questioned whether those who volunteer to augment the initial emergency medical response would have access to enough first-aid and basic medical supplies.

He indicated that the anatomy of a nuclear detonation can be dissected into blast, thermal, and radiation effects, each of which can cause significant injury.

Two types of blast forces occur simultaneously in the shock front of the nuclear detonation: (1) static overpressure effects measured in pounds per square inch (psi) over ambient pressure and (2) dynamic pressure effects (i.e., wind), measured in miles per hour (mph). Overpressure can cause eardrum rupture at a threshold of 5 psi and severe lung injury at 20 to 30 psi. However, blast winds are much stronger than hurricane winds, and can cause fragmentation and collapse of buildings and other objects, therefore creating flying debris (missiles) and projecting human bodies into the air, resulting in both penetrating and blunt trauma. The blast winds are significant because, for example, although 15 psi might rupture eardrums, the associated blast winds would be well over 300 mph and inflict serious injury and death (Glasstone and Dolan, 1977:Table 12.38; Alt et al., 1989:7; AFRRI, 2003:33-36).

Thermal radiation injury caused by the intense heat of the expanding fireball and thermal infrared radiation would result in first-, second-, and third-degree burns. The extremely bright flash of light from the detonation would cause a spectrum of blindness effects, ranging from temporary flash blindness to permanent total blindness, depending on the distance from and the visual orientation at the moment the nuclear device exploded.

Nuclear radiation injury would be caused either by the prompt radiation released immediately on detonation in the proximal blast zone or, if the detonation occurred at ground level, by exposure to radioactive fallout.

The magnitude of each of the blast, thermal, and radiation effects of a nuclear detonation would decrease substantially as a function of distance from the detonation site; but, depending on a number of factors, the consequences of a detonation, such as radioactive fallout, can still be far-reaching. Combined injuries are more likely to occur than a single type of injury from the prompt effects. Initial primary triage of combined injury patients should be based on conventional criteria of mechanical trauma and burns, because they are the primary cause of death in the first few days.

Removal of significant radiation contamination would occur simultaneously with the primary triage process. As data on the radiation dose became available, a secondary triage evaluation, now based on likely radiation injury, would be conducted after the first few days in such a mass casualty scenario.

After this introduction, Flynn introduced the two subject matter experts who spoke during this session. Brooke Buddemeier, a certified health physicist at Lawrence Livermore National Laboratory, reviewed the potential effects on the population in the immediate vicinity of the detonation and on the population in the downwind area covered with radioactive fallout. Cham Dallas, a toxicologist, chair of the Department of Health Policy and

Management and director of the Institute for Health Management and Mass Destruction Defense at the University of Georgia, then focused on the effects that a nuclear explosion would have on the capacity of the health care system in several of the Tier 1 UASI areas.

Health Effects

Introduction[6]

If a terrorist were to explode a 10-kt-equivalent IND at or near the center of a Tier 1 UASI city, at or near ground level, without warning and during a workday, the number of casualties needing immediate medical care would be very large. An even larger population would be at risk of exposure in the hours and days after the explosion to enough radioactive fallout to sicken or kill them unless they were able to quickly take appropriate steps to protect themselves (Figure 1).

It is not possible to predict the exact numbers of injured persons in such an event because, fortunately, there has never been a ground-level nuclear explosion in any city for comparison. As a result, there is no applicable experience to provide the insight and essential data required to formulate a detailed projection. Instead, models extrapolated from Hiroshima, Nagasaki, and nuclear bomb tests on Pacific atolls and in the Nevada desert more than half a century ago have been used to make estimates of the number of casualties. Clearly, these estimates are very rough for a number of reasons:

- As already noted, the Hiroshima and Nagasaki bombs that exploded were airbursts and therefore produced much less fallout than a ground-level detonation would.
- Atmospheric nuclear tests in Nevada had yields less than 100 kt, but most were detonated on top of steel towers 100 to 700 feet high. The few true surface shots were 1 kt or less "so that they provided relatively little useful information concerning the effects to be expected from weapons of higher energy" (Glasstone, 1977:419-420). The surface bursts in the Pacific Ocean tests drew large amounts of water into the cloud "so that the fallout was probably quite different from what would have been associated with a true land surface burst" (Glasstone, 1977:420).
- The test detonations were conducted in open terrain or ocean settings and not in the same topographical and structural circumstances or population densities of the Tier 1 cities being evaluated.
- The factors used to adjust for the moderating effects of buildings and local topography have been primarily ad hoc but can affect the results by factors of 2 or 3.

---

[6] This introduction to health effects was drafted by the committee.

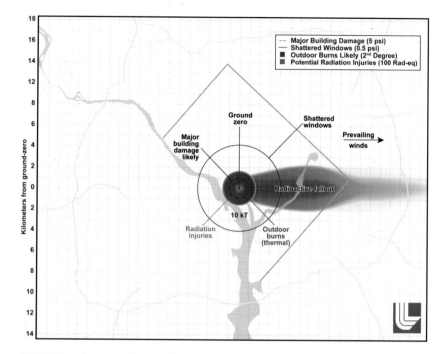

FIGURE 1 Sources of injury from a 10-kt IND: approximate blast, thermal, and prompt radiation effects around—and fallout effects downwind from—the detonation point.

SOURCE: Reprinted, with permission, from Lawrence Livermore National Laboratory, 2009. Copyright 2008 by Lawrence Livermore National Laboratory.

- Most models have calculated blast, burn, and radiation injuries separately and have not tried to determine the extent of combined injuries (i.e., estimates of blast, burn, and radiation injuries might count the same person as injured or killed two or three times).[7] Efforts are under way to produce improved human casualty estimates, but the work is in the early stages and the issue needs further study (see Box 1 and footnote 13).

The Nuclear/Radiological Incident Annex to the NRF states, "Even a small nuclear detonation in an urban area could result in over 100,000 fatalities (and many more injured), massive infrastructure damage, and

---

[7]An exception is a U.S. Army textbook, which estimates the percentages of the injured in a nuclear war by type of injury or combination of injuries (e.g., 40 percent from burns and irradiation combined and 20 percent from trauma, burns, and radiation combined) (Alt et al., 1989:Table 1-1).

BOX 1
Modeling the Effects of INDs in Modern U.S. Cities and
Implications for Response and Recovery Plans

The conference report on P.L. 110-28 of 2007 that directed DHS to sponsor the IOM workshop on the current level of medical readiness to respond to a nuclear detonation in Tier 1 UASI cities—summarized in this report—also directed DHS to model the effects of 0.1-, 1.0-, and 10-kt nuclear detonations in Tier 1 UASI cities and assess the capacity of current plans to respond to and recover from such effects. DHS assigned the nuclear effects modeling and response and recovery strategy analysis tasks to Lawrence Livermore, Los Alamos, and Sandia National Laboratories and established the Modeling and Analysis Coordination Working Group to oversee the effort.

The modeling results were used to identify key drivers in response planning and to assess and refine effective response strategies. A preliminary report on sheltering and evacuation strategies indicated that sheltering immediately after a detonation for a period of time is critical in reducing exposure to fallout, followed by informed evacuation ("informed" means that the location and intensity of the fallout area can be determined and communicated soon after the detonation) (Law et al., 2008).

A summary report of the modeling and response work is being prepared (Buddemeier and Dillon, forthcoming). It will provide guidance for response planning by summarizing the key factors to be considered in (1) developing a public protection strategy; (2) setting first responder priorities for protecting response personnel, assessing the regional situation, and protecting the public; and (3) avoiding common misperceptions about nuclear weapons and identifying critical issues in planning responses to an IND.

The modeling and response analyses also informed the effort by the Homeland Security Institute to develop a communications strategy for responding to a nuclear detonation in a U.S. city, also mandated by P.L. 110-28 (see Box 5 for an overview of that activity).

---

thousands of square kilometers of contaminated land."[8] That government estimate of effects from an IND detonation is very general, but it indicates that there would likely be more than 100,000 survivors with injuries that would have to be treated. Although this detail is not mentioned in the annex, it can be interpreted that many of the 100,000 fatalities might be those who live for weeks or possibly several months before succumbing to ARS, as described in the next section: Topic 2, "Medical Care of Victims of the Immediate and Fallout Effects of a 10-kt IND."

Several nonfederal experts have developed models of the effects that a nuclear explosion of approximately 10-kt yield would have in several U.S.

---

[8] See footnote 2 for a brief overview of the Nuclear/Radiological Incident Annex and its URL.

cities, using publicly available data and various government-developed fallout plume models. Those who assumed central business district explosions of approximately 10 kt in yield have estimated casualties (dead and injured) ranging from approximately 150,000 (Los Angeles) to 500,000 (New York City).[9]

Prompt (Immediate) Effects[10]

Brooke Buddemeier presented the health effects that could be expected to result from an IND detonation in Washington, DC, near the White House. His scenario is based on a 10-kt explosion during a workday, using the weather profile from May 23, 2005, when there was clear weather and prevailing winds were from the west. (See Box 2 for a summary of prompt effects.)

Blast Effects. The effects of the blast forces would damage or destroy most buildings within one-half mile of the detonation location and it is unlikely that most, if any, of the population in this area would survive.[11] From one-half mile to about a mile out, survival would most likely depend on the type of structure a person was in when the blast occurred. Even at a mile, the blast wave would have enough energy to overturn some cars and severely damage some light structures.

Those who survived building collapses would be subject to ruptured eardrums and injury from being thrown against solid objects or hit by flying objects. Missile injuries from broken window glass and other objects propelled by the blast wave may cause penetrating or blunt trauma for several miles. The number injured would depend on population density and the proportion of people who happened to be facing a nearby window at the moment of detonation.

In addition to the blast effects (in fact, preceding them), there would be thermal and nuclear radiation effects and flash blindness.

Thermal Radiation. Buddemeier said that past bomb tests indicate that about half of the people who are outdoors approximately one mile from—and in direct line of sight of—the detonation would receive potentially fatal third-degree burns. In Washington, DC, a daytime population of

---

[9] See, for example, Helfand et al., 2002 (12.5 kt in New York City); Bunn et al., 2003 (10 kt in New York City); Marrs, 2007 (10 kt in San Francisco); Ventura County, 2007 (10 kt in Los Angeles); and Uraneck, 2008 (10 kt in New York City).

[10] This section on prompt or immediate effects is based on the workshop presentation by Brooke Buddemeier.

[11] Small numbers of people in Hiroshima and Nagasaki within 500 meters of ground zero survived because at the moment of detonation they happened to be in basements or other locations that provided adequate protection from the initial effects.

BOX 2
Prompt Effects Summary

- Prompt casualties (injuries + fatalities) would include blast and burn effects, not just radiation exposure
  - "[M]issile injuries will predominate. About half of the patients seen will have wounds of their extremities. The thorax, abdomen, and head will be involved about equally."[a]
- Literature and models predict that
  - hundreds of thousands of casualties could occur from the prompt effects in the first few minutes within a few miles of detonation site,
  - the overall number of casualties is likely to be reduced by protection from the urban landscape and being within heavy buildings, and
  - tertiary effects (building collapse, glass and debris missiles, and flash blindness accidents) may increase the number of casualties.
- Those outdoors within a few miles could be blinded temporarily.
- Smoke, dust, and debris from the blast would cloud the air.

---

[a] U.S. Army. 1996. NATO *Handbook on the Medical Aspects of NBC Defensive Operations (Part I—Nuclear)*. Field Manual 8-9.
SOURCE: Adapted from the Buddemeier presentation at the workshop, June 26, 2008.

---

approximately 360,000 people would be within a mile of the hypothesized detonation point. However, relatively few people are outdoors during an average workday, and only a fraction of them would be in direct line of sight at the moment of the detonation. Modelers are working to account for such shadowing effects to determine the extent to which thermal effects would be reduced in modern U.S. cities.

Thermal radiation would also cause building fires that would be difficult to control and would increase the number of burn injuries. Fires would pose a special threat to survivors trapped in collapsed buildings.

Nuclear Radiation. Nuclear radiation effects would extend almost as far as the thermal effects. Anyone nine-tenths of a mile from the detonation who was unprotected by buildings or the terrain (i.e., in line of sight of the bomb) would receive a radiation dose of approximately 300 centigray (cGy) (see Box 3 for explanation of the centigray and its equivalence to other radiation units used in this report).[12] Almost every person exposed to this level would become ill and about half would die in the coming weeks

---

[12] The workshop presenters used different measures of radiation exposure and biological impact, including the cGy, rem, and rad. Box 3 defines these units and their equivalence and is provided for reference throughout the report.

BOX 3
Radiation Unit Equivalencies

The workshop presenters used different measures of radiation, including cGy, rad, and rem. The official internationally agreed-on SI (Système International d'Unités or International System of Units) units are the gray (Gy) and sievert (Sv), but the legacy units—radiation absorbed dose (rad) and roentgen equivalent man (rem)—are still widely used in the United States, in part because they are still used in current government regulations and guides dealing with radiation health and safety, such as the Environmental Protection Agency's (EPA's) *Manual of Protective Action Guides and Protective Actions for Nuclear Incidents,* issued in 1992. Even recent documents, such as the *Planning Guidance for Protection and Recovery Following Radiological Dispersal Device (RDD) and Improvised Nuclear Device (IND) Incidents* issued by DHS in August 2008 and the *Planning Guidance for Response to a Nuclear Detonation* issued by the Executive Office of the President in January 2009 use rem and rad units (although the SI equivalents are given in parentheses following each time rem or rad values are used).

Rad and gray measure the absorbed dose, which is the energy imparted by radiation to an absorbing material. However, for a given absorbed dose, such as 1 gray, radiation of one type has a greater biological effect than radiation of another type. The measure of the biological effect of an absorbed dose, called the dose equivalent, is measured in rem or sieverts. The dose equivalent equals the absorbed dose times a quality factor (QF). QF = 1 for gamma, x-ray, and beta radiation; QF = 5, 10, 20, or 30 for other types of radiation, such as neutron, proton, and alpha radiation.

Absorbed Dose

    1 rad = 0.01 Gy or 10 milligray (mGy)
    1 rad = 1 cGy
    1 Gy = 100 rad

Dose Equivalent

    1 rem = 0.01 Sv or 10 millisievert (mSv)
    1 Sv = 100 rem

Because QF = 1 for gamma radiation, the main constituent of fallout, rad and Gy are essentially equivalent to rem and sievert. Thus, for purposes of this report when describing the hazards of fallout:

    1 Gy = 1 Sv = 100 rad = 100 rem

SOURCE: NCRP, 2005.

---

and months in the absence of treatment or supportive care (Table 1). As with thermal effects, however, few people would be outdoors and in the line of sight of a detonation in a modern U.S. city, so the number of deaths would likely be substantially less than bomb tests conducted on relatively

TABLE 1 Estimated Acute Symptom and Death Rates from Radiation as a Function of Short-Term Whole-Body Absorbed Dose

Dose (rad [Gy])	Acute Death from Radiation Without Medical Treatment (%)	Acute Death from Radiation with Medical Treatment (%)	Acute Symptoms (Nausea and Vomiting Within 4 Hours) (%)
50 (0.5)	0	0	0
100 (1.0)	<5	0	5-30
150 (1.5)	<5	<5	40
200 (2.0)	5	<5	40
300 (3.0)	30-50	15-30	75
600 (6.0)	95-100	50	100
1,000 (10.0)	100	>90	100

NOTE: Acute symptom and death percentages are estimated for healthy adults. They would be higher for children and those with additional (i.e., combined) injuries. Most acute deaths would occur 1 to 3 months after exposure. Those who survived short-term radiation exposure would also be at higher lifetime risk of cancer, an issue that is mentioned but not addressed in this report.
SOURCE: NCRP, 2005 (for 2 Gy, EOP, 2009).

flat open land would indicate. Also, the effect falls off rapidly with distance. For example, at one mile, the estimated radiation dose would be 100 cGy, which might cause nausea and vomiting but not fatalities.

Flash Blindness. In addition to nuclear and thermal radiation, the detonation would create a brilliant flash of light that could cause temporary blindness to anyone outdoors up to more than 5 miles away. This effect could travel even farther if there is good visibility, if there are clouds to reflect the light, or if the event occurs at night. Flash blindness could occur even if the victim is not looking in the direction of the detonation. It can last several seconds to minutes. Although this effect does not cause permanent damage, the sudden loss of vision to drivers and pilots could cause a large number of traffic casualties and make many roads impassable.

Buddemeier concluded that current models are based on data from past nuclear events and provide predictions based on a flat plain in which all structures would be in line of sight of the detonation. Primary effects could cause hundreds of thousands of casualties in the first few minutes within a few miles of the explosion. However, the casualty reduction in a major city due to the protective effects of modern urban buildings is unknown. It is also difficult to be precise about the number of casualties because the mechanisms of how ground-level nuclear blast, radiation, and thermal effects propagate through the modern urban environment are not well understood. The extent of different combinations of injuries from various effects is also unknown but is thought to be substantial. In addition, secondary and tertiary effects, including flying glass and other missiles, building collapses, and flash blindness, are not well understood and may cause a significant number of additional casualties. For example, how many people within several miles of the detonation would happen to be near a window when the blast wave arrives a few moments later? How many drivers would be temporarily blinded by the flash or by thick clouds of dust and therefore crash their vehicles? The state of the weather and wind directions and speeds at the time of a detonation would also affect the number and types of casualties. Finally, the absolute number of casualties would also depend on the density of population, which varies substantially across Tier 1 UASI areas.[13]

Delayed Effects of Fallout[14]

In addition to the direct effects, a ground-level explosion, unlike the airbursts over Hiroshima and Nagasaki, would produce a substantial amount of radioactive fallout. This fallout would kill and injure a large number of people unless they were able to evacuate in time or take shelter where they were, preferably in a basement as far as possible from the radioactive debris that will have fallen on the ground and roofs. (See Box 4 for a summary of fallout effects.)

In a ground-level detonation, half the energy of the explosion is directed downward, into the ground. The vaporized and irradiated earth is pulled up into the fireball, which ascends rapidly into a towering mushroom cloud. The radioactive debris then falls back to the ground, beginning with the heaviest particles.

An area extending approximately nine miles downwind would be covered with enough fallout to pose an immediate danger to the life and health of emergency medical and other rescue personnel as well as to inhabitants who were outdoors for even short periods of time during the first several

---

[13] After the workshop, Buddemeier reported results of new modeling work performed at Lawrence Livermore National Laboratory on the effects of low-yield nuclear explosions, including the number and type of prompt injuries likely to result after taking into account the protective effects of buildings. The Washington, DC, scenario would result in approximately 250,000 people injured by blast, thermal, or radiation effects, or by some combination of the three. Of these, 100,000 would benefit most from advanced medical aid. Approximately 100,000 of the injured would probably recover without advanced medical aid, and 50,000 would succumb to fatal doses of radiation or combinations of injuries in the coming weeks and months. (Buddemeier did not provide an estimate of the number of prompt fatalities from blast, burns, or radiation.) The number of injured could be reduced by appropriate protective actions by the public, but the numbers also depend on population density. In New York City, for example, approximately 400,000 would benefit most from advanced medical care (Buddemeier, 2008:Slide 24).

[14] This section on delayed effects from radioactive fallout is based on the workshop presentation by Buddemeier.

BOX 4
Fallout Effects Summary

- The fallout cloud could climb 5 miles high and would be carried by upper atmosphere winds (often at high speeds).
- Hundreds of thousands of acute casualties from radioactive fallout could occur within an area extending about 9 miles downwind of ground zero.
- The number of fallout casualties could be reduced by action (i.e., sheltering or evacuation).
- Radiation levels decay rapidly with time.
- In the first few days, the primary health hazard is external gamma radiation from fallout on horizontal surfaces. Breathing in fallout dust is of less concern in the first few days and would not be a major contributor to overall exposure or immediate morbidity and mortality.
- Radiation has a delayed effect. Although radiation sickness may manifest within a few hours, victims of lethal radiation may not succumb for days or weeks.

SOURCE: Adapted from Buddemeier presentation at workshop, June 26, 2008.

---

hours. Areas further downwind would receive progressively less fallout but still pose a risk of ARS to anyone who spent enough time in the open. Even where there would not be enough fallout to cause acute injury, its long-term effects might lead to an increase in the rates of certain diseases (e.g., cancers, cataracts), an issue not addressed in this workshop. In Buddemeier's scenario, for example, approximately one million people could be exposed to a dose of 1 cGy or more if outside in the contamination for the first 4 days, which is the dose level at which taking protective action (sheltering or evacuation) should begin to reduce long-term effects, according to Environmental Protection Agency (EPA, 1992) and DHS (2008) guidelines.

Buddemeier emphasized the speed with which the fallout arrives after the moment of detonation. Radioactive debris and dust from a 10-kt explosion can reach a height of 5 miles and is quickly dispersed by high-speed upper-atmosphere winds. (On May 23, 2005, the day that Buddemeier used in his scenario, upper-atmosphere winds were measured at up to 75 mph.) The heaviest and therefore most dangerous particles of fallout would be on the ground for about 9 miles downwind within minutes. (In the Washington, DC, scenario, the fallout cloud would go on to reach Chesapeake Bay within 30 minutes and the Atlantic Ocean within 2 hours.)

Any person outside who was within 2.5 miles downwind of the detonation during the first 2 hours would receive approximately 600 cGy, a dose that without treatment would cause serious ARS and probable death. At

5 miles downwind, the dose would be 300 cGy, which would still cause ARS; the odds of death without treatment would be about 50 percent. At 9 miles, a person still outside after 2 hours would receive approximately 100 cGy, which could cause mild symptoms but not death. At 12 miles, the 2-hour accumulated dose would be down to 50 cGy, at which point radiation effects would probably be detectable but not life-threatening.[15]

Not only does fallout decrease sharply with distance, it also decays quickly with time. It is most dangerous in the first few hours after an explosion. More than half its energy is given off in the first hour and more than 80 percent in the first day.

In the scenario Buddemeier presented, the U.S. Capitol was 1.6 miles downwind of the explosion, in the middle of the fallout plume. Anyone going outside near the U.S. Capitol 15 minutes after detonation would receive ~1,500 cGy per hour. At that exposure rate a person could receive up to 200 cGy in 8 minutes. After the first 2 hours the dose rate would be down to 180 cGy per hour and it would take more than an hour to reach 200 cGy. Two days after detonation the dose rate would be down to 7 cGy per hour, at which 28 hours would be required to receive 200 cGy.

Based on his scenario, Buddemeier observed that individuals near an IND detonation would be making life-or-death decisions in the first few minutes or hours. They will be deciding: Am I better off sheltering or evacuating? If I take shelter, how will I know when it is safe to evacuate? Many people who were not near enough to be injured by the prompt effects of an IND detonation would still be at risk of injury from fallout beginning soon after the explosion. In most cases, the correct course of action to prevent or minimize injury from fallout would be to stay inside—or go inside immediately—because the fallout would be on the ground too soon to escape by fleeing.

Sheltering inside a building could provide substantial protection from radiation. For example, sheltering in the basement of a house would avoid between 90 and 98 percent (depending on the number of stories and construction) of the exposure that someone outside would receive. Sheltering in the core or basement of a large office building could reduce exposure by 99 percent or more compared with being outside (Figure 2).

Buddemeier concluded his presentation with several observations and recommendations. He observed that few state and local communities have a coordinated response plan for the aftermath of nuclear terrorism; there is a general lack of understanding of response needs; and there is uncertainty about federal, state, and local roles and responsibilities. He also observed

---

[15] For reference, the occupational dose limit for whole-body radiation is 5 cGy a year. A dose of 25-50 cGy would affect the bone marrow and reduce white blood cell counts but probably not cause symptoms. For the sake of comparison, the whole-body computed tomography scan delivers an effective dose of ~10 mSv (1 cGy).

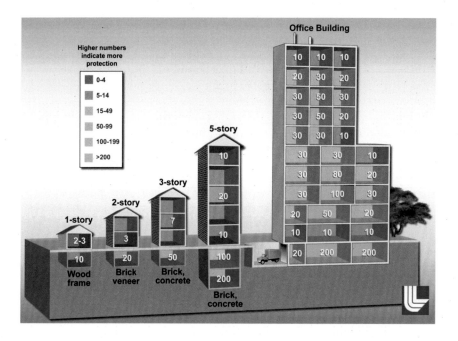

FIGURE 2 Protection from exposure to radiation provided by sheltering in different types of structures and various places within those structures.
NOTE: The numbers in this figure represent the protection factor (PF). Like the sun protection factor (SPF) for sunscreen, the higher the PF, the greater the protection. To obtain the sheltered exposure, divide the outdoor exposure by the PF. For example, a person on the top floor, periphery, or ground level of the office building pictured would have a PF of 10 and receive only one-tenth (or 10 percent) of the exposure that someone outside would receive. Someone in the core of the building several floors up would have a PF of 100 and receive only one one-hundredth (or 1 percent) of the outdoor exposure. Sheltering in the basement of the one-, two-, or three-story dwellings pictured would give a person 10, 5, or 2 percent, respectively, of the exposure that someone outside would receive.
SOURCE: Reprinted, with permission, from Lawrence Livermore National Laboratory, 2009. Copyright 2008 by Lawrence Livermore National Laboratory.

that decisions made in the first few hours have the greatest public health and medical impact. The impulse to evacuate might prove to be counterproductive in terms of minimizing radiation exposure and its health impact because, in most cases, the best way to reduce radiation exposure would be to shelter in place initially. Finally, he said there is a lack of scientific consensus on the most appropriate response strategies.

He recommended that the scientific community become more engaged in improving the basic understanding of a low-yield nuclear detonation in a modern city (e.g., by evaluating the efficacy of shelter and evacuation strategies, the type and distribution of injuries and public health infrastructure, the efficacy of response strategies, and the effects on critical infrastructure such as communications and electrical power systems). He further recommended that the federal government clearly define policies, provide guidance, and clarify its actions after a nuclear detonation in a U.S. city.[16] Finally, because response strategies to an IND detonation would be community-specific, preparedness tools and support adapted to local needs are required.

Effects on the Area Health Care System

Cham Dallas from the University of Georgia presented the results of work he did with his colleague William Bell on the effects of a 10-kt nuclear detonation near the White House, which had been presented at a hearing of the Senate Committee on Homeland Security and Governmental Affairs on April 15, 2008 (Dallas, 2008).[17] Using a model and data provided by the Defense Threat Reduction Agency, Dallas estimated that there would be at least 150,000 serious injuries, at least 70 percent of which could be fatal. He estimated that these numbers could be 4 to 8 times higher in more densely populated cities such as New York and Chicago.

Dallas also presented the results of modeling that he and Bell did specifically for the workshop concerning the number and distribution of injuries caused by a 10-kt explosion in Washington, DC, and other Tier 1 UASI cities. He simulated the various effects in each city within the circle in which the blast overpressure would be 0.6 psi or greater—the threshold for breaking windows.

Given his assumptions[18] and estimates of the workday population for the DC simulation, Dallas estimated that approximately 720,000 people would be in this circle in the Washington, DC, area, of whom approximately 105,000 would receive a radiation dose of 150 rem (1.5 Sv) or more from prompt radiation or fallout (an exposure sufficient to cause clinical

---

[16] In January 2009, after the workshop was held, a federal interagency committee under the auspices of the Homeland Security Council and Office of Science and Technology Policy in the Executive Office of the President released a 92-page *Planning Guidance for Response to a Nuclear Detonation* "to provide [state and local] emergency planners with nuclear detonation-specific response recommendations to maximize the preservation of life in the event of an urban nuclear detonation . . . for the first few days (e.g., 24-72 hours) when it is likely that many federal resources will still be en route to the incident" (EOP, 2009:7).

[17] See also Bell and Dallas (2007) and Dallas and Bell (2007).

[18] The assumptions were detonation at 20 meters and median September three-dimensional weather with clouds above the fireball.

symptoms in most people). (See Box 3 for explanation of the rem radiation unit and its equivalence to other radiation units used in this report.) Of the 105,000 people receiving at least this much radiation, approximately half would have received 680 rem (6.8 Sv) or more, which would most likely result in death no matter what treatment they received, and 5 percent would have received 150-300 rem (1.5-3.0 Sv), which they would probably survive without treatment. The remaining 45,000 would have received 300-680 rem (3.0-6.8 Sv) and would have only about a 50 percent chance of survival unless they received intensive treatment. Not all of these people would survive the other effects of the detonation, however. Approximately 16,000 would be in the area in which nearly every building would have been flattened by the detonation. On the other hand, others exposed to lower doses of radiation or no radiation at all would require treatment for serious and life-threatening blast and thermal injuries.

Dallas provided an admittedly rough estimate of the number of injured needing hospital care after a 10-kt event in Washington, DC—nearly 180,000—but did not do similar calculations for the other cities. The numbers would vary by city, however, because of differences in population density. In Dallas's model, for example, the number of people receiving 300-680 rem (3.0-6.8 Sv) within the 0.6-psi perimeter would range from approximately 42,000 in San Francisco to 460,000 in New York City.

Rather than trying to estimate the number of injured needing hospital care (except for Washington, DC), Dallas estimated the numbers of hospital beds that could be available within 4, 24, and 48 hours at various distances up to 300 miles from each city. According to his calculations, the only way to secure a substantial proportion of the beds likely to be needed would be to empty half of them within a 300-mile radius of ground zero within 48 hours. He also assumed that it would be possible to move thousands of patients up to 300 miles to fill all the freed-up beds, that enough hospital staff would report to work, that no hospitals would be closed due to fallout, and that there would be no additional detonation within the 300-mile radius.

In the case of Washington, DC, for example, Dallas estimated that approximately 5,000 beds would be available within 50 miles. After 24 hours, this number could increase to 12,000 within 100 miles. Given a best-case (some would say unrealistic) scenario that half the beds within 300 miles would be available 48 hours after the event, the maximum number of available beds would be at most 120,000, about two-thirds of the number of injured predicted by the simulation. In reality, the actual number would probably be less, given the difficulties of emptying filled beds, the likelihood of staffing shortages, and the lack of capability to move so many patients in 2 days.

Finally, Dallas looked at the effect on hospitals near the detonation points. In his New York City simulation, in which the detonation point is in midtown Manhattan near Rockefeller Center and the fallout plume goes over the southern end of the island, no hospitals would be in the zone of total destruction, a few would experience structural damage and possible casualties, and a total of 13 would be within the 1-psi perimeter and have most of their windows blown out. Two of the 13 would also experience dangerous levels of radiation from fallout (more than 300 rem [3.0 Sv] in one case, more than 530 rem [5.3 Sv] in the other). Five more of the 13 would receive lesser levels of radiation, as would two hospitals outside the 1-psi perimeter. The impact on the health care infrastructure in Washington, DC, would likely be less. In the specific scenario presented, only two hospitals would be in the 1-psi perimeter with none under the fallout plume. Far more problematic than the actual loss of hospitals, however, would be the inability to transport patients to receiving hospitals. Dallas deemed it highly unlikely that most patients could be moved in sufficient time through the chaotic environment following a nuclear detonation to distant hospitals in the unaffected areas. High traffic volume, fear instilled by uncertainty of the actual location of the radiation plume, and the intense clinical needs of burn victims, serious trauma patients, and radiation-exposed people would severely hamper patient transport.

In his summary, Dallas was not sanguine about the capacity of the health care system to care for the victims of a 10-kt IND detonation even under the most optimistic conditions (i.e., ability to fill half the hospital beds within 300 miles). During his presentation, he suggested that there would be a disproportionate need for eye care (because of broken glass and other missiles and retinal burns) and for burn beds. There are approximately 1,500 burn beds in the country, which are typically 80 to 90 percent full on any given day. He concluded with a list of factors affecting health care access in a 10-kt event:

- The number of individuals concerned that they might have been exposed who would go to medical facilities and seek evaluation
- The extent of transportation problems because of gridlock, rubble in the streets, damage to highways, loss of power to traffic lights, and other factors
- The availability of hospital security (a lack of security accounted for most of the hospital closures in the aftermath of Katrina)
- The number of accessible hospital beds and medical personnel willing and able to work
- The number of nearby and usable 3,000-foot runways to land C-130s for air evacuation[19]

---

[19] During another presentation, there was discussion of using railroads, which radiate from all urban areas, for evacuation of victims.

- The availability of rapid and effective screening tools for determining individual radiation exposures (these currently are not available, except in the most rudimentary forms, but are needed for treatment and are under development)

Discussion of Health Effects and Health Care System Impacts

The discussion following the presentations by Buddemeier and Dallas touched on several issues. One had to do with protective strategies. For example, would it be advisable to mandate sheltering to minimize radiation exposure and help keep highways open for rescue, security, and health care personnel? Some downsides of making sheltering in place the standard response were mentioned, including the potential threat from area fires set off by the detonation as well as differences in the proportions from city to city of houses with brick walls and concrete-wall basements versus single-story wood houses without basements that would be significantly less protective. Any one-size-fits-all policy would result in increases in risk for some individuals. Each individual would have to decide what to do, and the focus should be on improving that decision making. This requires more than people being well informed in advance so they are capable of deciding to stay or leave. It also requires a capability of getting information to them during a nuclear event about where the fallout is heading and where it is deposited, current rates of radiation, and other information (e.g., highway conditions).

Another question concerned how well the communications infrastructure would survive the electromagnetic pulse (EMP) generated by the detonation as well as the blast and thermal damage. For example, it would be useful to have a "reverse 911" capacity to inform specific areas of when it is safe to evacuate. Buddemeier explained that destruction of electronic equipment by the EMP from a 10-kt IND ground burst is probably not going to extend beyond the area already hit hard by the blast overpressure wave. In any case, hospitals and other organizations should have backup plans for communication failures, whatever the cause.

There was discussion of the Cold War attitude that it is useless to plan for a nuclear event "because we'll all be dead anyway." Several participants argued that low-yield INDs would be different. An IND explosion would still be catastrophic in terms of casualties, but many people not touched by the initial blast would be able to avoid or reduce exposure to injurious radiation doses stemming from the fallout if they knew what protective actions to take.

A participant wondered if plume prediction models would be accurate and fast enough to be useful in an actual event. Buddemeier stressed again how quickly the fallout deposition occurs, particularly in areas close to the detonation. In his view, the plume concept is somewhat problematic because it conjures up an image of a cloud overhead that one can escape by quickly evacuating. In fact, fallout heavy enough to cause acute injury could arrive too quickly to outrun. Planning for evacuation would be more feasible in areas farther downwind, where dose levels would be too low to cause acute effects but could induce cancer years later (e.g., Delaware would be affected, should there be an IND event in Washington, DC).

A participant asked if the infiltration of fallout particles in buildings was factored into the estimates of protection afforded by different types of buildings. Buddemeier said that this has been studied and the effect is minimal relative to the dose coming from the fallout lying on the surfaces outside. In any case, conventional planning would be likely to result in the shutdown of climate control systems in large buildings.

Flynn, a committee member, suggested using nontraditional means to increase health care system capacity. In austere conditions, retired nurses and doctors, and nursing and medical students, could work with medical teams. Technicians and nonmedical individuals could be trained to provide certain services, such as starting IVs, debriding burns, applying skin medication, and dressing wounds, all under some level of medical supervision, at least initially. Another participant discussed the need to educate physicians and other medical personnel about radiation so they would be more willing to work in its presence.

Another participant brought up the possible reluctance of jurisdictions across the country to lend response personnel to a city hit with an IND because of fears that they may be next. There also may be restrictions on air travel and movement of goods that could hamper the medical response.

Committee member Frederick Burkle pointed to the British approach to triage during the Cold War threat of the 1980s. They estimated that if London was hit by a 20-megaton bomb, each surviving physician would have a very large number (600-900) patients to treat. This would necessitate difficult and demanding triage decisions and reevaluation of the goals of triage. Therefore, the British trained volunteer government officials as triage management officers to take the burden of triage work off health care providers alone and refocused triage less on health and more on societal survival. A 10-kt detonation, however, would be less devastating (although still catastrophic), making it potentially possible to reduce the impact of casualties from fallout if an appropriate triage-management system was in place and proper resources were available.

Summary of 10-kt Detonation Effects

Detonation of a 10-kt-yield IND in the central business district of a large U.S. city would be catastrophic for most people within a few miles, but it would not kill or even injure most people in the city or metropolitan area. However, many people would be at risk of injury from radioactive fallout following the detonation unless they swiftly took appropriate protective measures.

The number of casualties caused by the immediate effects of the explosion is difficult to determine. The protective shielding afforded by modern office buildings is not well understood, although it is probably significant. The number of people who would be killed and injured from the combined effects of blast, thermal radiation, and prompt radiation is also not well understood. Tertiary effects such as missile injuries, building collapses, flash blindness, and broken windows would increase casualties, but by how much is not known.

If an IND was detonated at or near ground level, as seems most likely, a substantial amount of fallout would be created and deposited over a large area. Fallout that would be radioactive enough to expose anyone outdoors to lethal doses would be deposited for about 9 miles downwind. Moreover, this fallout would be deposited rapidly, making evacuation dangerous. Beyond 9 miles, the dose rate from fallout would decrease but still might have potential health consequences for anyone who was outside for many hours or—farther out—for several days. Even when the dose fell too low to cause acute effects no matter how long the exposure, the probability of long-term effects, such as cancer, would extend for about 250 miles.

In areas of intense fallout, sheltering on the first floor of a typical house or, better yet, in the basement, could reduce the dose by a factor of 5 to 100. The dose rate falls off exponentially with time, however, so in many cases it would be safe to evacuate from what had been a high-dose area after the first few hours.

Although a 10-kt IND detonation might not destroy or disable many hospitals (depending on the detonation point and the prevailing winds), the number of beds in any major city or even its metropolitan area relative to the number injured would be inadequate. Even if one was able to empty half the beds for 300 miles around and transport patients that far—very optimistic assumptions—there still would not be enough beds, especially critical care and burn beds.

For medical and public health planning purposes, it would be prudent to assume that there would be thousands to tens of thousands of people injured by the prompt effects of the explosion, in addition to those killed outright. Some would have traumatic injuries from the effects of the blast wave (e.g., fractures, lacerations, organ damage), some would have serious thermal injuries (e.g., flash burns from the explosion, flame burns from fires started by the explosion), and some would have both. Many of the same people would have received doses of ionizing radiation sufficient to sicken or kill them. The combination of these injuries—thermal and traumatic injuries—significantly increases the overall severity and potential lethality of any additional radiation exposure that the individual might have experienced. Some number of people who did not have blast or thermal injuries would have received clinically significant doses of radiation. Even people with high doses of radiation would not become seriously ill for days or weeks, but they should be identified early so they can be sent to facilities able to provide the supportive care they will need to survive the period of bone marrow suppression and other effects caused by radiation.

There would be many eye injuries, both retinal burns in those who happened to be facing the detonation point and injuries from shattered window glass. An unknown number of people would be injured in vehicle and other types of accidents caused by temporary blindness from the flash of the detonation.

For medical and public health planning purposes, it would also be prudent to expect anywhere from tens of thousands to more than one hundred thousand injuries from radioactive fallout, although this number could be greatly reduced if there were advance preparations for mass evacuations and sheltering in place and if there were effective means for providing people with the information they could use to reduce their exposure as much as possible.

Because of the anxiety a detonation would produce, health system planners should also expect a large number of unexposed individuals to want to be screened for radiation exposure. Although most of those in fallout areas would not have received high enough doses to cause acute radiation sickness, many would have received low, subacute doses. This population, which could be more than one million people, would need to be identified and assigned to long-term follow-up for radiation-induced cancers, which would probably occur among them at a higher rate than normal in the years to come.

Finally, planners should consider the impact of a detonation on the capacity of the health care system to respond. There would likely be many more casualties than the emergency medical services (EMS) and hospitals in or near the affected city could handle. In any case, planners should anticipate that some responders may themselves be victims and that some nearby facilities may be degraded or damaged. Hospitals might have been hit by the blast, or exposed to fallout, or be short of personnel, or all three situations may have occurred. Some responders and health care providers would be victims themselves, and others might be deterred from working by the prospect of radiation exposure or be preoccupied with evacuating their families.[20]

---

[20] Research on attitudes of first responders and medical personnel toward reporting to work after an incident involving radiation is reviewed by Becker under Topic 5, "Risk Communication, Public Reactions, and Psychological Consequences in the Event of a 10-kt IND Detonation."

TOPIC 2: MEDICAL CARE OF VICTIMS OF
THE IMMEDIATE AND FALLOUT EFFECTS
OF A 10-kt IND DETONATION

After reviewing the results of simulation models of the effects of a 10-kt IND detonation on human health and health care systems and after hearing order-of-magnitude estimates of the number of casualties, the workshop turned to a review of the state of the art in treating victims of nuclear explosions and radioactive fallout. John Mercier, a health physicist and director of military medical operations at the Armed Forces Radiobiology Research Institute (AFRRI), presented the U.S. military's approach to treating prompt casualties with combined injuries in the event of a nuclear attack and discussed how to adapt it to the civilian setting. Fred Mettler, a committee member and chief of Radiology and Nuclear Medicine at the New Mexico Federal Regional Medical Center, presented the state of the art in caring for fallout casualties (i.e., treating ARS).

John Mercier began with a quick review of the effects of the atomic bomb exploded over Hiroshima. There were 136,000 casualties, about half the population. Approximately 25,000 to 30,000 died the first day. After 4 months, the death toll was 64,000, leaving 72,000 injured. About 70 percent (50,000) of the injured had combined injuries (i.e., radiation combined with trauma or burns) from the blast, thermal, and prompt radiation effects. (There was very little fallout because the bomb was detonated in the air.) The health care system was badly damaged. Only 3 of the 45 hospitals were functional, and their windows were blown out. More than 90 percent of the physicians and nurses were casualties (some kept working despite significant injuries). The injured reached hospitals on their own or with the aid of friends and neighbors.

In the military, Mercier said, the medical guidance in a mass casualty event is based on the reality that resources will not be sufficient to provide standard treatment to everyone, and it might be necessary to follow altered standards of care. The military mass casualty guidance for austere situations (i.e., when there are inadequate resources for the patient load and alternate standards of care are necessary) is as follows:

1. Provide the maximum care for the maximum number of patients.
2. Determine if it would be more effective to move hospitals to the impacted area to free up limited patient evacuation assets.
3. Determine methods for rapid evacuation of patients to tertiary care centers that can provide appropriate care.
4. Conserve limited medical resources:
    - Those expected to live have the highest priority for resources, but provide comfort care to those expected to die.

- Avoid procedures that would reduce any patient's ability to care for himself or herself.
- Do not use trained medical personnel for first aid or rescue operations. Train all nonmedical personnel and rescue teams in first aid (applying dressings, controlling hemorrhages, applying field splints, handling the injured).
- Perform only the most expedient treatments sufficient to meet immediate medical requirements of the patient. Use only simple bandages, splints, etc., needed to stabilize patients for evacuation.

Triage is the key to effective management of a mass casualty event, military or civilian. The Department of Defense (DoD) uses the DIME system for triage, in which the patient priority categories are Delayed, Immediate, Minimal, and Expectant. A similar system, Simple Triage and Rapid Treatment (START), is widely used in the civilian community to sort casualties into categories:

- Those needing *immediate* attention
- Those for whom treatment of life-threatening but potentially treatable injuries can be *delayed*
- Those who have *minimal* injuries
- The *expectant*, that is, those who will die despite treatment

Using START (or the pediatric version, JumpSTART), triage can be performed in one minute per patient using an algorithm to check respiration, perfusion, and mental status.

No triage system currently exists that satisfies the requirements faced in a nuclear disaster. Thus, the use of such triage may be problematic in a nuclear event, because victims may have survivable traumatic injuries if treated but will be inevitably doomed by their radiation injuries. Furthermore, the mortality rate at any given dose level of radiation is higher if the radiation is combined with mechanical trauma, burns, or both.

Currently there is no adequate field test to establish the dose of radiation a person has received. This makes it difficult to determine who will eventually die despite medical treatment. Knowing who is in the expectant category would make it possible to focus limited personnel and resources on victims who would have a better chance of surviving if they received early medical attention.

The only—and very rough—indicators of radiation dose for initial triage in the field are the location of the victim relative to the detonation point at the time of detonation; time to onset and severity of nausea, vomiting, and diarrhea; and clinical symptoms and signs (such as early presence of skin erythema). Of these, time to vomiting is the most reliable, although still imperfect, indicator of radiation dose.

Mercier presented a triage algorithm with adjustments in the triage categories for radiation dose. For example, persons without trauma or burns who received a low dose (less than 200 cGy) would require only ambulatory monitoring. If an otherwise uninjured person received a dose of 200 cGy or more, ambulatory monitoring would be followed by routine care and eventual hospitalization, if clinical symptoms and blood counts warranted. However, anyone in the delayed triage category for trauma or burns who was judged to have received a dose of 200 cGy or more would be shifted to immediate. Similarly, anyone categorized as immediate for trauma or burns who received more than 600 cGy would be shifted to expectant. Victims who reported vomiting within an hour of the attack would be considered to have been exposed to more than 600 cGy; those vomiting between 1 and 4 hours after the attack would be assigned an estimated dose between 200 and 600 cGy; and those vomiting more than 4 hours after the attack would be assigned less than 200 cGy.[21]

If a radiation event involved one person or a few people, even with mechanical trauma or burns from the detonation of a dirty bomb, for example, there would be no need to triage. No one would be labeled expectant, even those with estimated doses of 1,000 cGy or more. In this situation everyone could receive standard care without overly burdening the health care system. Trauma and burns could be treated as part of the normal patient load of emergency departments (EDs) and patients could be placed in intensive care or transported to tertiary care facilities for specialized care as the individual's circumstances required. Laboratory tests could be performed to estimate the radiation dose, determine prognosis, diagnose ARS, and manage treatment of ARS (including dicentric chromosome assays, which only a limited number of laboratories in the country can perform).[22]

---

[21] HHS introduced the Radiation Event Medical Management (REMM) website (http://www.remm.nlm.gov) in March 2007 as guidance on diagnosis and treatment for health care providers. REMM also includes triage categories with modifications for combined injury, although the radiation dose cutoffs are somewhat different. This guideline would move anyone in the immediate or delayed categories with a radiation dose larger than 450 cGy to the expectant category to receive comfort care. It would shift anyone in the delayed category for trauma to immediate if the radiation dose were between 150 and 450 cGy. Those without any trauma or burns who received doses of 150 cGy or larger would be given ambulatory monitoring with routine care in a mass casualty situation, although in a non-mass-casualty setting they would be hospitalized until their bone marrow was back to normal (http://www.remm.nlm.gov/radtrauma.htm, accessed June 23, 2009).

[22] The dicentric chromosome assay is the "gold standard" biodosimetry method for radiation dose assessment (Prasanna et al., 2008). Unfortunately, in addition to being limited in availability, the assay takes several days to perform, which also limits its use in a mass casualty situation.

Hospitals would provide intensive, individualized supportive care for all persons with significant exposures.

In his presentation, Fred Mettler emphasized that ARS does not manifest itself immediately. The onset of ARS may occur within a day or two in people exposed to extremely high doses for which death is 90 percent likely or higher (830 cGy or more). But the latent phase can extend for days or weeks in victims whose doses would probably be survivable with intensive care (300-530 cGy).

Thus, for patients primarily afflicted with radiation injury (i.e., without major trauma or burns), the effects requiring medical attention and resources would not present immediately but would evolve over several weeks after the IND is detonated. The task of the early medical response will be to identify those who will require delayed care for ARS. The assessment necessary to make such determinations includes the following:

- Taking careful medical histories that document where a person was relative to the detonation point (e.g., how far away, how long outside and when, in what kind of structure, and how long) and when he or she may have vomited
- Performing a physical examination to document signs and symptoms affecting the hematopoietic, gastrointestinal, cerebrovascular, and cutaneous systems
- Drawing a series of blood samples over time to track lymphocyte depletion
- Possibly drawing a single blood sample for dicentric chromosome analysis, if necessary and if resources permit

Performing clinical assessments of several hundred thousand people within the first several days after an IND explosion would obviously pose tremendous challenges. The main goal is to determine who would benefit from supportive medical care (essentially those receiving total body doses between approximately 200 and 800 cGy).

If there were just one or a few cases of radiation exposure, the victims would be hospitalized until they recovered and receive individualized evaluation and treatment. In a mass casualty situation, however, victims who have received radiation doses that would normally hospitalize them (200 cGy or more) might be examined and then assigned to outpatient monitoring and routine care, unless their condition worsened and they required hospitalization.

Mettler also stressed that, although radiation levels of fallout may decay quickly (enough in several days to enable someone to leave the area after sheltering in a basement or building without suffering much additional exposure dose), the fallout is still on the ground and the dose still accumulates over time. He cited the example of a bomb test at Bikini Atoll in the Pacific Ocean that exposed Marshallese villagers on nearby islands to fallout. In the first 4 days, the villagers received an average of 220 rad (2.2 Gy). By the end of a year, they had received 180 more on average, for a total average of 400 rad (4.1 Gy) (see Box 3 for explanation of the rad unit and its equivalence to other radiation units used in this report). He cited similar statistics from the villages around Chernobyl. He also briefly discussed the long-term implications of radiation exposure, although this topic was outside the scope of the workshop except to the extent that early actions would be needed to identify the exposed so they could be tracked for decades.

Another point made by Mettler concerned the variability in the deposition of fallout because of shifts in wind direction. The wind at 5,000 feet (the top of the fallout cloud from a 10-kt detonation) may be going in a completely different direction than the wind at the surface, which not only complicates the deposition pattern but also makes it difficult to know which way to evacuate to escape exposure to fallout. The likely patchwork pattern of fallout due to varying wind patterns over time and at different altitudes means that millions of people will need to be tested for exposure.

Finally, Mettler noted that, from a public health point of view, appropriate protective action taken by individuals to avoid or reduce irradiation would save many times more lives than medical treatment of the same people if they did not act to reduce exposure. He suggested focusing plans for responding to an IND event on efforts to minimize radiation exposure as the best investment.

Discussion of Medical Care of Victims of a Nuclear Detonation

A workshop participant expressed his concern that medical personnel might require excessive decontamination of patients before treating them. He suggested that if the standard were two times the background level of radiation, for example, people with serious trauma would die unnecessarily. Mercier agreed that life-threatening injuries should be treated before definitive decontamination. Mettler noted that removal of clothing will reduce contamination substantially. A further level of decontamination could be readily achieved by simple rinsing with a cloth or sponge or by showering.

Another concern expressed was how to resupply medical facilities in the affected metropolitan area. Many hospitals maintain only a day's supply of drugs to reduce inventory costs and therefore depend on daily deliveries of supplies. Both speakers agreed that this should be an important part of planning a medical disaster response. Mercier noted that in most cases of radiation exposure, patients do not become neutropenic within the first week and may not need a transfusion or support with other blood products for the first 2 weeks or so or longer, depending on the dose they received. This does not apply, however, to patients with combined injuries who need immediate trauma care.

Several participants were skeptical that people would take orders to shelter in place or to evacuate. Mercier cited studies finding the rate of shadow evacuation in disasters (i.e., self-evacuation regardless of government direction) to be 30 to 40 percent. There was some discussion of how to make the government's message more effective.

Committee member George Annas noted that DHS expects that the public will strongly resist leaving personal items (e.g., wallets, keys, purses, pictures, jewelry) behind in the contaminated zone. He asked if confiscating wallets and purses at mass decontamination sites was necessary or advisable. Everyone who commented agreed that it was neither advisable nor necessary, because the amount of radiation on these items would be minimal and, in any event, the contents of the wallets and purses would be shielded from radiation by being inside of them. Mettler also noted that self-decontamination at home would be easy and very effective if people knew what to do. This could also decrease the numbers at mass decontamination sites, and permitting people to keep their valuables would make the entire process much more efficient and user-friendly.

A participant wondered how the civilian sector could learn more from the defense sector about medical preparedness for nuclear events. Mercier said he and others participate extensively in interagency activities addressing this issue, but military experts on nuclear preparedness are a shrinking pool, far fewer than 20 years ago. AFRRI has been partnering with the National Institutes of Health (NIH), universities, and pharmaceutical companies on developing medical countermeasures.

Finally, a participant pointed out that the expectant casualties will also need palliative or comfort care. This will require resources, although less than trauma care and supportive care for ARS. It was suggested that the Strategic National Stockpile (SNS) should include morphine and other palliative medicines for people with ARS who are not expected to survive.

TOPIC 3: EXPECTED BENEFIT OF RADIATION COUNTERMEASURES

This session of the workshop did not address all the medical countermeasures that will be needed in the event of an IND attack. For example, better treatments for combined injuries of explosions will be needed, but they were not discussed because the charge to the committee was only to evaluate the efficacy and expected benefit of *radiation* countermeasures, both those currently available and those under development.

Richard Hatchett, the member of the committee who moderated this session, began by summarizing the current situation. Licensed radiation countermeasures are currently available, but they are specific to radionuclide or isotope. No drug is licensed for the treatment of ARS at this time. However, several effective therapeutics (e.g., reparative cytokines, such as granulocyte colony-stimulating factor, granulocyte-macrophage colony-stimulating factor, and keratynocyte growth factor) are currently available and could possibly be used "off label" by attending physicians. Also, a number of very promising candidate drugs for ARS are currently in the research and development (R&D) pipeline. There is no proven or Food and Drug Administration (FDA)-approved antidote for irradiation received from external sources after exposure, only supportive treatments to help victims survive the acute effects caused by the radiation.

Hatchett laid out the three most important challenges in his view to the development of radiation countermeasures:

1. Identifying drugs that work
2. Getting these drugs licensed
3. Delivering these products to people who need them

Also in this session, Albert Wiley, director of the Radiation Emergency Assistance Center/Training Site (REAC/TS) of the Department of Energy (DOE), reviewed currently available medical countermeasures. Nelson Chao, head of cell therapy at Duke University and principal investigator for one of the NIH Centers for Medical Countermeasures Against Radiation, reviewed products currently under development. Carmen Maher, who is in the Office of Counterterrorism and Emerging Threats at FDA and a U.S. Public Health Service commander, described the policy and procedures for approving emergency use of medical products that are licensed for treating ARS. Steven Adams, deputy director of the SNS program of the Centers for Disease Control and Prevention (CDC), talked about the logistical challenges of delivering medical supplies and equipment in a post-detonation environment.

Albert Wiley began by reviewing radiation countermeasures that are currently available to treat internal contamination by radioisotopes. He did not discuss supportive treatments, such as antibiotics, antivirals, antifungals, cytokines, and stem-cell transplants, because it is highly unlikely that such medications would be required for acute deterministic effects in organ systems such as bone marrow that would occur from inhalation of fission products. He emphasized that other public health measures to avoid radioactive materials, such as sheltering or evacuation, are better ways to reduce acute radiation exposure from internal contamination when compared with currently available medical countermeasures.

At this time, medical countermeasures act on and reduce exposure only from radionuclides that have entered the body through inhalation, ingestion, skin, or open wounds. Radionuclides may contaminate the airway or the gastrointestinal system, or they may be taken up or incorporated into cells, tissues, and organs. In the case of an IND detonation, contamination and incorporation might occur from inhaling fission products as the fallout cloud descended, from resuspension of fallout on the ground, or from ingesting water or food contaminated with fallout.

The spectrum of hundreds of fission products produced from an IND detonation would vary depending on whether it was an air or ground burst and whether the weapon is enriched uranium- or plutonium-based. Some of the medically important products include iodine-131, cesium-137, strontium-90, cobalt-60, plutonium-239, and uranium-235.

Decorporating and blocking agents are very specific to the nuclide involved. Most of the countermeasures work by hastening the elimination of the nuclide from the body in urine or stool, by blocking its uptake, or both. The treatment for tritium, for example, is to drink 3 to 4 liters of water a day to dilute and help excrete it. Prussian Blue can be used to bind with cesium-137 in the gastrointestinal tract so that it cannot be absorbed and will interrupt the normal hepatoenteric cycle, thus enhancing its fecal excretion. Zinc- and calcium-DTPA (diethylenetriamine pentaacetic acid) are chelating agents that work by binding to plutonium-239 and to other actinides (e.g., americium, curium) to enhance their excretion in the urine. Potassium iodide (KI) blocks uptake of iodine-131 by the thyroid.

The SNS includes KI, Prussian Blue, and the DTPAs. While Wiley did not estimate the probabilities of internal contamination from an IND explosion that would require administration of these countermeasures, the earlier presentation by Buddemeier explained that the most dangerous fallout for producing acute injury consists of large particles that fall quickly to the ground and are not respirable. These particles produce radiation that may injure the skin and other organ systems from external contamination, whereas internalized radionuclides are unlikely to pose a short-term danger to the population in the area of the fallout.

Consequently, for several reasons, the aforementioned decorporating and blocking agents will not be a high priority in the immediate aftermath of an IND detonation. Most people in a position to inhale fallout would already be much more severely affected by the external exposure from fallout on the ground around them. If they were inside, protected from external radiation, the risk of internal contamination would also be greatly reduced. If they did inhale these larger particles, they would not present much of a hazard, because the upper nasopharynx would trap most of the larger particles and then they would be coughed up, expectorated, or swallowed. Wiley noted that the more serious internal contamination hazard is posed by soluble radionuclide compounds that would eventually contaminate water and food, but he mentioned that this is a problem that would be addressed by EPA and the U.S. Department of Agriculture after the initial response to the explosion.

A radiation spectrum analysis is necessary to identify specifically these internalized nuclides. Further clinical management would then rely on laboratory testing of urine and stool as well as whole-body or lung radiation detectors/counters. DTPA must be administered intravenously in a clinical setting. Medical facilities overwhelmed by trauma and burn cases and patients with high-dose exposures will not likely have the staff or resources to provide chelating and decorporation agents. Finally, FDA-approved decorporation, blocking, and other medical countermeasures exist for only a portion of the radionuclides present in fallout.

Wiley then concluded that the necessity to use current FDA-licensed radiation countermeasures (i.e., the decorporating and blocking agents Prussian Blue, zinc- and calcium-DTPA, and KI) for the treatment of internalized radionuclides would be largely academic during the first days after an IND detonation, because the external doses would be so much larger than the dose from internalized radionuclides. Initially, medical responders would be preoccupied with treating the immediately life-threatening physical trauma and burn injuries.

Some of the current countermeasures are, however, routinely and effectively used to reduce the stochastic risk associated with radionuclide intakes from industrial and laboratory accidents, and they would be useful in reducing stochastic risks in populations that have inhaled plume radionuclides associated with radiological dispersal device (RDD) scenarios.[23] In these scenarios, the numbers of casualties would be lower and specific nuclides for which there are countermeasures would be more likely to be present. Also, while the acute casualties are being cared for, some of the current countermeasures would be useful in reducing the organ or tissue doses associated with ingestion of radionuclides in contaminated water and food in the initial days following an IND detonation.

Nelson Chao reviewed potential novel agents that promise to mitigate the effects of radiation. The effects include

- hematopoietic ARS, in which bone marrow suppression causes neutropenia, thrombocytopenia, anemia, and lymphopenia;

---

[23] The word stochastic means "random" or "by chance." In the context of radiation, *stochastic* risk usually refers to the probability that any given individual in a population exposed to low-level ionizing radiation will incur cancer, often years later. Most scientists assume that there is no threshold dose for the stochastic effects of low-level radiation. For a stochastic effect the degree of malignancy is unrelated to dose. In contrast, *deterministic* risk is the probability of incurring an acute effect, such as ARS, which occurs above a certain threshold dose of radiation and the severity of the effect is proportional to the dose.

- gastrointestinal ARS, where serious injury to the intestinal tract leads to prolonged severe nausea, vomiting, diarrhea, ulceration of the intestinal mucosa, and systemic infection leading to sepsis;
- lung injury, in which individuals who survive initial hematopoietic and gastrointestinal injury develop radiation pneumonitis and fibrosis, with initial symptoms developing 2 to 3 months after exposure;
- kidney injury;
- cutaneous radiation syndrome; and
- radiation combined injury.

Currently, the options for the treatment of ARS are limited. They include supportive care to prevent opportunistic infections, control of gastrointestinal symptoms (e.g., antibiotics, antivirals, and antifungals), cytokines to stimulate bone marrow, and mitigation of skin toxicity. Cytokines are not approved by FDA for victims of a radiological attack, but they could be administered off label and they must be administered on an individual basis under the supervision of a physician. This, however, would be exceedingly difficult to accomplish with mass casualties and overloaded medical facilities. In cases with high levels of exposure to radiation, patients would require the support of critical care or intensive care to survive the period when the blood-forming capacity of their bone marrow has failed. The availability of critical and intensive care beds would be problematic in a mass casualty situation (see, e.g., Rubinson et al., 2008).

Chao outlined a rational strategy for identifying and developing potential agents currently used by the Centers for Medical Countermeasures Against Radiation, eight extramural cooperative research centers that have been funded by NIH since 2005. The strategy—built on decades of earlier R&D from DoD, DOE, and the radiobiological science community at large—is to use the pathophysiologic processes leading to hematopoietic and gastrointestinal ARS to identify points of intervention on which to focus research and development (Table 2). Chao's view is that the area in which improvement would save the most lives is the prevention or reversal of the hematopoietic effects in patients who have received enough radiation to suppress their bone marrow significantly but not enough radiation to cause death from gastrointestinal toxicity.

Chao reviewed the status of some of the countermeasures under development and some of the research findings concerning efficacy. Some agents are being readied for FDA-required animal efficacy studies. These include agents already licensed by FDA for other uses, such as human growth hormone, granulocyte colony-stimulating factor (filgrastim and pegfilgrastim), and granulocyte-macrophage colony-stimulating factor (sargramostim). Some are in Phase III clinical trials for other indications, such as certain thrombopoietin-receptor-activating peptides (to counter

TABLE 2 Treatment Strategies for Hematopoietic ARS

Pathophysiologic Process	Intervention
ROS-induced injury	ROS scavengers, antioxidants, and cytoprotective agents
Committed precursor depletion	Nutrients, growth factors, and antiapoptotic agents
Stem cell depletion/stromal damage	Modulators of cell death (MSCs, EPCs)
Cytopenias	Immunomodulators, cytokines, and endothelial-oriented interventions
Immunological compromise	Reconstitution of immunity
Bacteremia, fungemia, viremia	Antibiotics, antifungals, and antivirals
Adverse tissue remodeling	Antifibrotic strategies

NOTE: EPC = endothelial progenitor cells; MSC = mesenchymal stem cells; ROS = reactive oxygen species.
SOURCE: Presentation of Nelson Chao at the workshop, June 26, 2008; he also presented a parallel table of treatment strategies for gastrointestinal ARS.

radiation-induced thrombocytopenia[24]), mesenchymal stem cells (to treat gastrointestinal ARS and cutaneous radiation syndrome), and pirfenidone (to prevent radiation-induced fibrosis of the lung). Others are being readied for Investigational New Drug status so that they can be tested in clinical trials. Yet others are undergoing basic pre-clinical testing, including novel cell therapies, such as endothelial cell transplantation and myeloid progenitor cell transplantation.

Carmen Maher said FDA's mission includes facilitating the development and availability of medical countermeasures to the effects of WMDs. Currently there are no FDA-approved drugs for ARS.

FDA has several regulatory avenues to help speed the approval of medical countermeasures, including

- fast-track designation for certain products;
- priority reviews of certain products;
- accelerated approval through surrogate markers, which are laboratory measures of biological activity within the body that indirectly indicate the effect of treatment on disease state; and
- the animal efficacy rule, which allows approval or licensure of a product based on animal efficacy data when human efficacy studies cannot be conducted.

---

[24] Since the workshop, two such products—romiplostim and eltrombopag—have received FDA licensure for another indication, idiopathic thrombocytopenic purpura.

In addition, FDA can approve an emergency-use Investigational New Drug application at the request of a licensed clinician for a specific patient, usually for products either undergoing clinical trials or for which the clinical trials have just been completed. FDA also has a treatment-use Investigational New Drug application, which is for expanded access or wider use. The limitation on these regulatory options is the stringent Investigational New Drug rules, including informed consent, approval by an institutional review board (IRB), patient follow-up, strict recordkeeping, and careful data collection requirements. They also allow only for either single-patient use or for use in specific populations. They are suited for clinical research studies but would be administratively burdensome at best, and needlessly restrictive at worst, in public health emergencies with mass casualties.

To address the FDA-approval issue with many promising WMD medical countermeasures, the Project Bioshield Act of 2004 amended Section 564 of the Food, Drug, and Cosmetic Act to allow emergency use of medical products during a declared emergency involving a heightened risk of attack on the public or U.S. military forces or a significant potential to affect national security. The Emergency Use Authorization (EUA) provision allows the commissioner of FDA to approve emergency use of unapproved products or unapproved uses of approved products (Nightingale et al., 2007).[25] The procedures require

- a declaration of emergency by the secretary of the Department of Health and Human Services (HHS), based on a determination by the secretary of Homeland Security that there is a domestic emergency involving a heightened risk of attack to the U.S. population with a chemical, biological, radiological, or nuclear (CBRN) threat agent, or a determination by the secretary of Defense that there is a military emergency involving a heightened risk of attack to military forces with a CBRN threat agent, or a determination by the secretary of HHS that there is a public health emergency involving a CBRN threat agent that affects, or has the potential to affect, national security;
- a request from someone outside FDA for an EUA;
- consultation (to the extent possible under the circumstances) by the commissioner of FDA with the directors of NIH and CDC; and
- a conclusion by the commissioner of FDA that
  - o the CBRN threat agent specified in the emergency declaration can cause a serious or life-threatening disease or condition;

---

[25] FDA's "Guidance: Emergency Use Authorization of Medical Products" is at http://www.fda.gov/oc/guidance/emergencyuse.html (accessed June 23, 2009).

o   it is reasonable to believe, on the basis of the totality of
    scientific evidence available, that the medical product may
    be effective (i.e., there must be some evidence to support the
    intended use of the product);
o   the known and potential benefits of the medical product
    outweigh the known and potential risks; and
o   no adequate, approved, alternative medical product is
    available.

Maher noted that legally FDA cannot issue an EUA in advance by, for
example, pre-authorizing use of a product if and when a certain type of
emergency occurs. There must be an emergency declaration by the secretary
of HHS for an EUA to be issued by the FDA commissioner.[26]

The SNS includes FDA-approved products. Prussian Blue, for example,
could be shipped to a locality hit by an IND detonation because it is
approved for a specific population. But an EUA would have to be authorized before Prussian Blue could be used in children under 2 years old
because it is not approved by FDA for that age group. Similarly, filgrastim
is in the SNS, and it could be delivered to and used legally by hospitals
that have run out of filgrastim for their hematology and oncology patients.
However, it is not indicated by FDA for use on victims of ARS without an
EUA, because it is not approved for treatment of radiation casualties.

A declaration of an emergency—and with it, any associated EUA—is
in effect for 1 year. The EUA may be revoked earlier if, for example, there
are data indicating that the product is doing more harm than good, or
the product is not making a difference, or the criteria for issuance cease
to exist.

HHS has established an Emergency Use Authorization Working Group.
The EUA working group is an interagency committee consisting of federal
officials with expertise in public health, medicine, law, ethics, and risk communication that recommends uses of EUAs to the secretary of HHS and
the commissioner of FDA. The most recent time that the EUA process was

---

[26] Subsequent to the workshop, however, in October 2008, FDA approved a request from
the Biomedical Advanced Research and Development Authority at HHS for an EUA for the
pre-event provision and potential use of doxycycline hyclate tablets in emergency kits for
inhalational anthrax, to be provided to United States Postal Service (USPS) participants in
the postal module of the Cities Readiness Initiative (CRI) and their household members. The
request was based on a September 23, 2008, determination by the secretary of Homeland
Security and an October 1 declaration by the secretary of HHS that there is a significant
potential for a domestic emergency involving a heightened risk of attack with *Bacillus
anthracis,* the causative agent of anthrax. (The CRI postal module involves the delivery of
antibiotics to residences in selected zip codes by USPS participants where there may have been
an intentional release of *Bacillus anthracis.*)

followed in a large-scale exercise was TOPOFF (Top Officials) 4.[27] In that case, it took approximately 10 hours from the time that FDA received the EUA request to the time that the EUA was issued.

Steven Adams described the SNS. It currently contains about $3.8 billion of medical materiel—antibiotics, medical supplies, antidotes, antitoxins, antivirals, vaccines, and other pharmaceuticals. Part of it is contained in 12 "push packages" located in strategic locations around the country; the push package can be transported from these locations to one of the pre-arranged "receipt, stage, and storage" (RSS) sites in each state within 12 hours of a decision to deploy the SNS. This transport would be accomplished by commercial partners (e.g., Federal Express and United Parcel Service) using either air or ground movement. The federal decision to deploy SNS assets is made by the secretary of HHS and follows a request by the affected state's governor and an evaluation of the situation by HHS, CDC, and other federal officials.

Once the push package (which consists of 130 air freight containers totaling about 50 tons) arrives at an RSS, the state is responsible for breaking it down and transporting the contents needed to the affected locality or localities. Each locality is then responsible for delivering the contents to hospitals, other medical care facilities, or mass dispensing points from which they can be distributed. Along with push packages, the SNS program could rapidly deploy a small technical advisory team to assist state and local officials with medical logistical issues.

The push packages contain enough medicines and other medical supplies to supplement the initial local response. The SNS program can also draw on much larger reserves of managed inventory, which are designed to be delivered to the state by ground or air within 24 to 36 hours.

At this point, the SNS has modest amounts of the cytokine filgrastim along with other supplies relevant to an IND event. They include bandages and dressings; intravenous administration supplies; fluid and electrolyte resuscitation; airway maintenance and management supplies, including ventilators; antimicrobials, antivirals, and antifungals; burn care; pain management and sedation; anti-emetics; and trauma and wound care products.

---

[27] The U.S. Congress, responding to terrorist events such as the 1995 attack on the Tokyo subway with sarin gas, concluded in 1998 that U.S. top government officials should receive better training to respond to a complex attack involving WMDs. To address this challenge, Congress mandated the Department of State and the Department of Justice to conduct a series of challenging, role-playing exercises involving the senior federal, state, and local officials who would direct crisis management and consequence management response to an actual WMD attack. The result was TOPOFF, a national-level domestic and international exercise series designed to produce a more effective, coordinated, global response to WMD terrorism (http://www.state.gov/s/ct/about/c16661.htm, accessed June 23, 2009).

Adams listed a series of challenges in responding to an IND explosion. The SNS program assumes that, because of the size and extent of disruption created by an IND detonation, medical materiel should be pushed forward immediately to the vicinity of the explosion, rather than held back pending specific requests. The SNS might be able to deliver supplies and a cadre of technical advisers to an airfield 30 miles outside the detonation zone, but it will be up to others—presumably people who are already there—to move it to where the supplies are needed. The challenges include

- the probability that the critical local staff involved in planning and implementing the response will be out of commission;
- a loss of infrastructure of all types;
- a shift of responsibility for the medical and public health response to surrounding jurisdictions not hit by the blast or fallout;
- the disruption of communication, affecting situational awareness and command and control even if the infrastructure is intact;
- the displacement of population through "shadow migration" (i.e., not ordered by authorities) in the early hours before people can be informed whether they should be moving or sheltering where they are to protect themselves;
- the potential for disruption to civil authority; and,
- absent reliable individual dosimetry, the need to triage and treat based on presumptive estimates of the amount of radiation a victim has received.

Discussion of Radiation Countermeasures

The importance of colony-stimulating factors, such as filgrastim, in the mass casualty treatment of radiation injury—and the steps needed to use it—were discussed further. Maher explained that filgrastim could be delivered as part of the SNS, but using it to treat radiation injury from an IND detonation would make it an Investigational New Drug for that purpose.[28] In this situation, an EUA would be the best mechanism for gaining approval of its use because it would not entail informed consent and an IRB, although patients would have to be told that the filgrastim was being given under an EUA and have the right to refuse it. In terms of the SNS, Adams said the request for delivery of the stockpile must come from the state, through the governor's office. The basis for the request should be that local capacity has been exceeded. A participant noted that there is a workaround in that situation. Because filgrastim, sargramostim, and other cytokines are licensed products, they can be used off label by community physicians. If hospitals

---

[28] Filgrastim is only approved by FDA for treatment of cancer patients experiencing severe neutropenia from chemotherapy or of patients with severe chronic congenital, cyclic, or idiopathic neutropenia.

had stocks of cytokines for licensed indications, they could be used off label in accordance with the recommendations of multiple groups, including the SNS Radiation Working Group.[29] A participant urged the SNS program to move the stockpile immediately in an IND event, in anticipation of emergency FDA approval of off-label use of products in the stockpile.

Maher added that FDA has a pre-EUA process in which data supporting the effectiveness of, for example, filgrastim for lethal levels of radiation in animals may be submitted and thus be in hand in the event of an IND detonation to support an EUA at that point.

There were mixed views of the need for KI. Iodine-131 is volatile and most of it produced in a nuclear detonation—as opposed to a reactor accident—would stay in the atmosphere for a long time. On the other hand, some people, including children and pregnant women, could receive 30 or 40 cGy to the thyroid, which would put them at risk of developing thyroid cancer in future years.

There was discussion of how many days after exposure that the administration of cytokines would be effective. Evidence from animal studies indicates that the effectiveness after a week could be zero. The current consensus opinion is that cytokines should be used within 2 or 3 days of exposure to radiation. Early administration of cytokines within 1 to 3 days following the IND detonation is clinically preferable.

TOPIC 4: PROTECTIVE ACTIONS AND INTERVENTIONS IN THE EVENT OF A 10-kt IND DETONATION

If a 10-kt IND were to detonate in a major U.S. city, there would be many unavoidable casualties from the prompt effects of the explosion itself. There would still be time, however, to avoid or reduce injuries from the residual levels of radiation around the detonation point and from fallout deposited downwind. The area immediately around ground zero would be too radioactive for rescue workers to enter, but the radiation dose rate would fall off steeply with distance and with time. There would be opportunities for saving lives in the ring of damaged buildings and building fires outside the zone of total destruction, but working in this area would expose rescue workers to lesser but still high doses of radiation. Doses above 5 rem (50 mSv) would increase the workers' long-term risks of cancer. Doses above 50 rem (500 mSv) would begin to elicit acute effects in some individuals as well as pose higher, dose-dependent probabilities of inducing cancer. At the time of the workshop, DHS had issued interim guidelines on emergency responder dose limits in an RDD or IND event and was working to finalize

---

[29] See Waselenko et al., 2004.

them (DHS, 2006). The guidelines did not impose a top limit on exposure, leaving it to incident commanders and first responders to decide whether the risks incurred would be outweighed by the benefits of saving lives or preserving critical infrastructure in a high-radiation environment.

In this part of the workshop, Sara DeCair, a health physicist in the Center for Radiological Emergency Preparedness, Prevention, and Response at EPA presented EPA's rules and guidances on radiation exposure and discussed their applicability to an IND event. John MacKinney, deputy director of Nuclear/Radiological/Chemical Threats and Science and Technology Policy in the DHS Office of Policy Development, discussed the work of an interagency committee on protective action guidelines for RDDs and INDs. Jill Lipoti, director of the Division of Environmental Safety and Health in the New Jersey Department of Environmental Protection, gave a state perspective on protective actions. Eric Daxon, a health physicist at Battelle's San Antonio operations outlined the decision making situation of an incident commander in the field when considering the appropriate use of protective action guides (PAGs).

Sara DeCair first described worker protection standards, which are promulgated by the Nuclear Regulatory Commission (NRC), by the states for x-ray technicians and other occupations, and by the Occupational Safety and Health Administration (OSHA). NRC and OSHA limit occupational exposure of workers to 5 rem (50 mSv) per year (see Box 3 for an explanation of the rem and its equivalence to other radiation units used in this report). EPA's *Manual of Protective Action Guides and Protective Actions for Nuclear Events* (EPA, 1992), known as the PAG Manual, provides guidelines for protecting members of the public by evacuation, sheltering, or relocation, as well as guidelines for emergency workers. (It should be noted that the manual specifies that the PAGs apply only in incidents "other than nuclear war.")

According to the PAG Manual, protective actions for the public would usually be taken when the projected dose to individuals would be 1 rem. Sheltering could begin at even lower levels because it is relatively low cost and low risk compared with evacuation.

The guides, recognizing the public health and welfare impacts of a radiation release, provide higher limits for emergency responders. In these instances, higher exposure may be justified for a lifesaving operation or if the collective dose to a large population is significantly larger than the dose to the emergency workers. For example, the worker guideline for protection of critical infrastructure is 10 rem (100 mSv) if a lower dose is not practicable. The worker guideline for lifesaving or for protection of large populations is 25 rem (250 mSv). The latter guide could be even higher than 25 rem if it is a voluntary action of a person fully aware of the risks involved. (The PAG Manual contains two tables of information on the risks of higher exposures for workers contemplating volunteering to work in a radioactive zone, one on the short-term health risks of various high-dose levels received in a few hours, and the other on the long-term risks of cancer after exposure to 25 rem in a few hours.)

EPA has also developed "turn-back" rates of up to 10 Roentgen (0.00258 Curies per kilogram) per hour for protection of critical infrastructure in the early phase of a release. These conservative guides are more applicable for EPA's post-event cleanup responsibilities than for response to an IND event. DeCair noted, for example, that the fire departments in the National Capital Region have adopted 10 Roentgen per hour as defining a radioactive zone and 200 Roentgen (0.0516 Curies per kilogram) per hour as the absolute turn-back rate.

John MacKinney heads the DHS efforts to issue guidance for response to RDD or IND events. In his presentation he said that, while there is no dose limit for lifesaving actions, any actions resulting in doses higher than OSHA's 5-rem (50-mSv) annual limit must be voluntary. He mentioned two decision points. First, at projected doses higher than 5 rem the volunteer must understand the increased long-term risk of cancer with increasing dose. Second, if the projected dose is higher than 50 rem (500 mSv), the volunteer must understand the potential for acute effects as well as the increased cancer risk. In addition, the incident commander must be confident that the benefit of the mission outweighs the risk to response workers and, in the case of lifesaving, have confidence that there are victims who can be saved.

MacKinney gave some examples of situations in which the public benefit of exposing someone to high levels of radiation may be justified. Students may be sheltering in the basement of a school building in a radioactive zone. If the building were to catch on fire, exposure to high radiation long enough to put the fire out may be worthwhile. Or water pressure may be dangerously low in an area in which there are fires or a risk of fires, but a valve key to restoring it may be in the radioactive zone. A key issue, he pointed out, is properly estimating the radiation dose likely to result from a mission. Therefore, sufficient good-quality radiation data are critical to response operations planning. Responders also must have dosimeters and know how to use them. Incident commanders need training to know the health effects of different doses, and responders who volunteer also must understand them.

There will be an area around the detonation point, for example, between the 1- and 5-psi limits, in which there are likely to be survivors and radiation may be relatively low (e.g., opposite the direction of plume movement). The chance of having survivors lessens as physical damages increase with proximity to the detonation point. At overpressures above 5 psi, few survivors are expected. There may be much lifesaving to be done in areas that are not very radioactive in the 1- to 5-psi range. (In Buddemeier's Washington, DC, scenario, the highest dose level—i.e., under the center of the plume—would fall to less than 100 cGy beyond a mile from the detonation point.)

DHS published an interim RDD/IND guidance in 2006 (DHS, 2006) and is about to publish the final version.[30] The interim guidance was developed to apply the 1992 EPA PAG Manual to acts of terrorism. The EPA PAGs were developed to apply to the most likely nuclear incidents at the time, of which the most serious would have been a nuclear power plant or transportation accident. They were not designed to deal with radiological or nuclear terrorism.

The working group that developed the interim guidance determined that the existing PAGs for the early and intermediate phases published in the EPA PAG Manual are also appropriate for use in RDD and IND incidents. However, the interim guide recognizes that, in an IND event, decisions would have to be made much more quickly and with much less information than in a nuclear power plant event to be effective. More important, the EPA PAGs were recognized as inadequate to address the very-high-dose-rate zones and the extensive physical impacts of a nuclear explosion. A follow-up effort specific to nuclear response planning was promised.[31]

In the early phase, according to the interim guide, exposure of emergency workers should be limited to 5 rem (50 mSv) to the extent possible, and the population should be told to shelter or evacuate if the projected dose is between 1 and 5 rem (10 and 50 mSv). In the intermediate phase, workers should not be exposed to more than 5 rem per year, and the public should be relocated from areas in which the projected dose is 2 rem (20 mSv) or more during the first year.

Jill Lipoti began her talk by observing that the approach that would save the most people from injury and death in the event of an IND detonation would be sheltering for a period of time and then evacuating. She predicted that convincing people to shelter in place would be difficult and that the rate of self-evacuation, even in areas not directly impacted by

---

[30] The final version, *Planning Guidance for Protection and Recovery Following Radiological Dispersal Device (RDD) and Improvised Nuclear Device (IND) Incidents,* was issued on August 1, 2008 (DHS, 2008), and is summarized in the section "Summary of Protective Action Guides" in this report.

[31] The follow-up effort resulted in a document, *Planning Guidance for Response to a Nuclear Detonation,* which is summarized in footnote 16.

radioactivity, would be high due to perception of the radioactive hazard. In the long run it would probably also be difficult to convince people to return to an area that has been contaminated by radioactivity, even though the dose rate has fallen to a level deemed safe by officials, unless there has been active involvement by stakeholders in developing the "safe" level.

The desire to save the lives of people exposed to high doses of radiation must be balanced against the costs to the responders. Responders will want to do something to help, even if it means risking their lives. However, the number of casualties should not be increased by the incautious exposure of emergency responders to unacceptably high doses of radiation. This is compounded by the long-term risk from radiation exposure. The emergency responder would not experience immediate symptoms but would increase the risk of eventually incurring cancer. The appropriate radiation level that is acceptable to an emergency worker in terms of higher risk of contracting cancer is not clear.

Lipoti also listed a number of issues that must be addressed in cleaning up and recovering from an IND detonation, although these were not in the scope of the workshop. Cumulative long-term exposure would be a major risk, and solutions palatable to elected officials and their constituencies would not be purely technical. They would inevitably involve trade-offs with economic and political factors. Currently, an integrated framework for compiling data from environmental monitoring, assessing risks from likely exposure routes, identifying options for protective actions or mitigation, and reaching decisions based on stakeholder input does not exist.

Eric Daxon studies ways to improve the decision making of military field commanders in the stressful environment of a nuclear event. Like civilian incident decision makers, commanders are not usually health experts, but they are required to make decisions that balance the radiation health risks and nonradiation health risks with the benefits of a course of action. For radiation, this decision is complicated because for doses greater than 25 rem (250 mSv), the risk is a potential increase in the risk of cancer much later in life. Currently, there is no defensible method for comparing an increased risk of cancer with the nonradiation risks and the health benefits of the proposed action. In this instance, rather than being guidance, the PAG limit becomes a fixed number not to be exceeded rather than a flexible guide as intended.

Daxon called for more detailed guidance that would provide decision makers with the ability to directly compare the radiation health risks with nonradiation health risks and the health benefits of a proposed action. This is relatively straightforward for acute radiation effects (e.g., acute radiation syndrome, radiation burns), but complex for the long-term, increased cancer risk. This guidance would provide the decision maker with the ability to defensibly balance radiation health risks and nonradiation health risks with the benefits of the proposed action. Such a direct comparison would also facilitate explaining the decision rationale and defending the decision to stakeholders both during and after the event.[32]

Discussion of Protective Actions and Interventions

Fred Mettler, a committee member, mentioned an IOM report done at the request of the military on battlefield criteria for operating in radiation environments. That IOM committee could not give an absolute dose limit, in part because the long-term risks of cancer should be considered along with other short- and long-term risks. The report recommended training about long-term risks so that commanders on the ground are aware of them when they make decisions that also involve many other, more immediate factors (IOM, 1999).

There was discussion of the importance of responders having adequate dosimeters. In the aftermath of the Chernobyl accident, dosimeters quickly maxed out, but workers kept working and did not know what doses they ended up receiving. Having digital readout dosimeters available in the SNS was suggested.

Whether EMS or hospital personnel would report for work was discussed. Surveys indicate that significant percentages (60 percent in one study) would not show up because they were concerned about radiation, chose to stay home with children, or were evacuating their families (Qureshi et al., 2005; Cone and Cummings, 2006; Veenema et al., 2008; Chafee, 2009). This problem could be mitigated with education and training.

The discussion turned to the question of sheltering or evacuating (or sheltering and then evacuating). Should sheltering be the default guidance in advance, given that communications might be disrupted? The 1992 EPA PAG Manual has shelter and evacuation guidance and factors to consider, but the worst scenario contemplated was a nuclear power plant accident. States and localities with nuclear power plants have plans in place for sheltering and orderly evacuation. The population likely to be affected is probably aware of these plans, may have KI in hand (KI is most effective if taken before exposure and must be taken within hours of exposure to have any significant effect), and usually has some advance notice of a release. In an IND event, upward of a million people might be in the 1-cGy or higher fallout area, which could extend several hundred miles downwind. Only the population far from the detonation might possibly have enough time to evacuate before

---

[32] It should be noted that the National Council on Radiation Protection and Measurements outlines key elements of preparing emergency responders for nuclear and radiobiological terrorism (NCRP, 2005).

the fallout arrived. Even this assumes an ability to predict where the fallout cloud will go, a capacity to inform people of the situation, and plans in place to facilitate evacuation and avoid a situation where people are stuck in their cars for hours when they could be better protected from radiation by sheltering where they live or work. MacKinney and DeCair, who were part of the interagency effort to develop the RDD/IND guidance, said the guideline to shelter or evacuate at 1 to 5 rem (10 to 50 mSv) would not apply within the near-in radioactive zone. (In the Washington, DC, scenario, this would be the area extending about a mile around the detonation point and the area covered with fallout about 10 to 15 miles downwind during the 24 hours following the explosion.) There is no single best option—whether sheltering in place or evacuating—for everyone.

Also, if the detonation is sufficiently above ground level, there may be little or no fallout and no need to evacuate or shelter since fallout depends on if and how much the fireball hits and vaporizes the ground, sending dust into the air where it can pick up radiation and create the fallout.

Daniel Flynn, a committee member, suggested that a national registry be established of everyone who is capable of utilizing a Geiger counter and has access to one—for example, radiation-related physicians, health physicists, and radiation technologists at hospitals, nuclear power plants, and universities—who would be willing to volunteer in the event of a nuclear detonation, for example, by accompanying emergency responders and by assisting at patient collection points and triage sites, decontamination sites, population shelters, hospitals, and evacuation points.

Summary of Protective Action Guides

DHS has issued guidelines developed by an interagency committee for RDD and IND events (DHS, 2008). They are discretionary, not regulatory. During the initial and intermediate phases of the event (i.e., from the time of detonation until the cleanup phase days to weeks later), they suggest sheltering or evacuation for any people whose projected dose would be 1 rem (10 mSv) or more if they remained outside during the earlier phases following the IND detonation. The guidelines note that evacuation has health as well as economic costs when compared with sheltering, and they say that sheltering could begin as early as when the projected dose is 0.1 rem (1 mSv). For emergency responders, the guidelines suggest doses of no more than 5 rem (50 mSv) in the initial phase except in "exceptional circumstances" and no more than 5 rem in subsequent phases no matter what the circumstances. Exceptional circumstances are defined as those in which the public benefit, such as saving large populations and protecting critical infrastructure, outweighs the private costs to the responders of a heightened, albeit small, cancer risk (up to 25 rem or 250 mSv) or acute effects plus heightened cancer risk (at more than 25 rem). Also, responders must be fully informed of the risks and volunteer to expose themselves to the projected dose.

There were concerns that the information about projected doses would not exist in the hours or even days after an IND detonation and also that, given the magnitude of such an event, the decision points of 5, 10, and 25 rem (50, 100, and 250 mSv) would not be realistic and would be ignored in practice. Some participants thought the decision points were appropriate but more detailed guidelines for applying them are needed. Having some of the same concerns, the RDD/IND working group led by DHS is continuing work on protective action guides and recommendations applicable to the zones closest to the detonation point.[33]

TOPIC 5: RISK COMMUNICATION, PUBLIC REACTIONS, AND PSYCHOLOGICAL CONSEQUENCES IN THE EVENT OF A 10-kt IND DETONATION

The effectiveness of the medical response to an IND detonation would depend to a large extent on the appropriate swift actions of individuals, families, and small groups in the immediate aftermath of a devastating explosion and the associated radioactive fallout. Survivors near the detonation point where radiation levels are high would be deciding whether to flee or to stay inside for a few days until radiation levels became sublethal or lower. Emergency responders would be deciding whether it would be safe to try to rescue victims around ground zero who have traumatic injuries. Health care personnel would be deciding whether to report to work or to evacuate or shelter with their families.

Individuals not affected by the immediate effects would be deciding what to do about the fallout hazard and would likely be considering whether to escape in their vehicles or by some other method or to shelter in place. If separated from their children, they would likely be trying to reunite with them and wondering what to do after they are reunited, including whether to leave the area or to shelter in place for several days while awaiting further guidance.

The decisions about how best to react would be made in the face of uncertainty regarding the location and extent of radiation effects after a detonation. As a result, the number of individuals concerned about exposure and desiring to be tested would greatly increase.

There would also be uncertainty about which health care facilities were operating and, of those, how overloaded they were. In addition, there would be uncertainty about whether escape routes were still open.

---

[33] The working group reported in January 2009. See Footnote 16.

Decisions would also be greatly affected by the degree of understanding that people—including emergency responders, health care personnel, and the public—have about radiation effects. Such understanding would include knowledge about the health effects of different dose rates and total doses, the efficacy of different types of shelters in moderating the dose, and the exponential rate of decay of radioactivity over time. A lack of understanding or a misunderstanding of radiation effects could lead to overreaction or underreaction.

Committee member Robert Ursano, the moderator of this workshop session, introduced the session with a review of the behaviors of relevance and what is known about them from studies of previous disasters. He identified disaster preparedness, response, and recovery behaviors and noted that research has clarified our understanding of such behaviors in recent years.

Preparedness behaviors involve the planning that people do for an event and the preparations for carrying out the plan (e.g., developing a family evacuation plan or stocking a basement shelter with supplies). These behaviors are shaped by public education campaigns and by effective risk communication.

Response behaviors include evacuation and sheltering to minimize exposure to radiation. They also include going to health care facilities to be checked for radiation exposure. Other behavioral phenomena include "convergence" (i.e., individuals or groups who travel to the disaster area to help, whether out of curiosity, to locate surviving relatives, or for other reasons) and migration (i.e., a population who leaves the disaster area for good). Public officials who want to direct residents to evacuate or to shelter in place will find that compliance will not be 100 percent and will depend in part on the public understanding of the risks. A substantial share of those who did not evacuate from the New Orleans region before Hurricane Katrina could have gone but refused to leave (while the others did not have the means to leave).

Concerning recovery behaviors, the goal of terrorists is not just to inflict death and destruction but also to induce terror throughout the nation. Terrorists aim to erode our sense of national security, disrupt the continuity of society, and destroy the morale, cohesion, and shared values of the nation. Fear would produce stress, which would cause mental health casualties. There would be an increase in the incidence of psychiatric disorders (e.g., generalized anxiety, panic, posttraumatic stress disorder [PTSD], depression), psychological distress (e.g., insomnia, irritability, feelings of vulnerability, work absenteeism, withdrawal, social isolation), and health risk behaviors (e.g., smoking, imbibing alcohol, drug use). For example, the incidence of mental illness in the New Orleans area had doubled

5 to 8 months after Hurricane Katrina (mild to moderate mental illness from 10 to 20 percent and serious mental illness from 6 to 11 percent). The rate of mental disorders among rescue workers at the 1989 DC-10 airplane crash in Sioux City, Iowa, was 40 percent after 13 months; among rescue workers at the Oklahoma City Murrah Federal Building bombing in 1995, it was 38 percent after 34 months.

In the remainder of the session, Steven M. Becker, associate professor of public health at the University of Alabama at Birmingham, presented the results of studies of how the public, emergency responders, health care workers, and public health officials may respond in an IND event. H. Keith Florig, senior research engineer at Carnegie Mellon University, discussed risk communication and decision making in planning for and implementing responses to an IND detonation. Ann Norwood, senior associate at the Center for Biosecurity of the University of Pittsburgh Medical Center, addressed the psychological effects of an IND event in the affected community and its hospitals and also the likely effects in the rest of the country. Dori Reissman, senior medical advisor of the Office of the Director at the National Institute for Occupational Safety and Health, addressed the psychological impacts of a catastrophic event and its effects on how people are likely to behave as a result.

Steven M. Becker opened his presentation with the statement that "effective risk communication is central to the success or failure of efforts to manage any disaster." Timely, consistent, accurate, and comprehensible messaging is vital in order to

- provide people with appropriate protective action information;
- reduce deaths, injuries, and illnesses;
- prevent responses that may impede efforts to manage the incident;
- reduce psychological and social impacts; and
- help maintain public trust and confidence.

Becker noted that effective communication and emergency messaging would be especially challenging in an IND event. The detonation could occur without warning, there would be massive destruction and extensive injuries and loss of life, and there would likely be fear of additional attacks. Furthermore, emergency messaging would need to start immediately to save lives. This would be very important for populations in the path of fallout from the nuclear detonation. Finally, the fact that the event would involve radiation would further increase the communication challenges. Risk perception research has consistently shown that radiation is one of the most feared of all hazards, and emergencies involving radiation can produce high levels of apprehension and alarm. This fear of radiation can affect how a population reacts or responds to an IND incident, particularly when emergency information is limited or confusing (Slovic, 2001; Becker, 2007).

The 1979 Three Mile Island nuclear accident provides a case in point. For every person who was advised to evacuate, 45 people actually left the area. Ultimately, some 150,000 people fled. Concerns about potential exposure can also translate into large numbers of concerned people seeking examinations or care. In 1987 in Goiânia, Brazil, discarded medical radiotherapy equipment containing cesium chloride contaminated 249 people; 8 developed ARS, and 4 died. Because of widespread concerns about potential exposure, a staggering 112,000 people ultimately sought testing. Finally, uneasiness about radiation can also result in social stigma and discrimination against people and products from an affected area.

Preventing or reducing such impacts depends, in part, on providing people with the information they need and want, and doing so clearly and in a timely fashion. Becker reported on recent research on people's concerns, information needs, and preferred information sources in relation to a radiological or nuclear event (Becker, 2004). The work, which was funded by CDC, was linked to a larger effort to improve emergency message development for unconventional terrorism threats (Wray et al., 2008). To understand communication issues in a radiological/nuclear terrorism event, a total of 30 focus groups were conducted with 285 participants drawn from multiple U.S. regions and a variety of population groups (including ethnic minorities, urban and rural residents, those for whom English is a second language). In addition, a series of focused interviews was carried out. As part of the study, participants reviewed public information materials and protective action information. Among the key findings were the following:

- People's main concerns center on health issues. Thus, for communications to be most effective, they should focus on health concerns and be delivered (at least in part) by spokespersons and/or agencies with high credibility on health issues.
- In areas where people are accustomed to natural disasters (e.g., hurricanes, tornadoes), television meteorologists were seen as a trustworthy source of information because they were viewed as familiar and apolitical.
- Consistent with other research, substantial resistance was found to the idea of sheltering. Most often, the resistance stemmed from people's desire to immediately gather their children from school.
- Fatalistic attitudes about surviving a nuclear event clearly exist in the population, especially in minority populations. This is important and requires special attention, since fatalism can translate into a reduced likelihood that people will undertake protective actions.

- Some key protective action terms, such as "shelter in place," are not always clear to people and may be subject to multiple interpretations. Such terms need to be either explained better or replaced.

Becker also reported on research carried out with emergency responders regarding their concerns, information needs, and preferred information sources in a radiological or nuclear terrorism event. Nearly two dozen focus groups were carried out with first responders and first receivers (Becker, 2004, 2009). Among the main findings were the following:

- Emergency responders of all types have a high level of dedication to duty.
- At the same time, incidents involving radiation are seen as new and unfamiliar, and there was more concern and uncertainty about appropriate responses than for other agents and scenarios (including chemical and biological agents).
- There was also serious concern about the state of individual and organizational preparedness for radiological and nuclear incidents.

Nine of the focus groups were carried out with public health professionals. A key finding was that public health professionals are committed to helping but are often uncertain about their role in a radiological or nuclear emergency.

The most recent research was with hospital ED clinicians (Becker and Middleton, 2008). A series of focus groups was carried out at urban, rural, and suburban hospitals in three U.S. regions. The research found that the biggest concerns of physicians and nurses included

- the expectation that health care facilities would be overwhelmed by people worried about radiation exposure;
- ensuring the safety of the health care workers' own family members;
- uncertainty as to whether portions of the staff would report for duty because of concerns about their own safety, the safety of their families, or both. This is consistent with surveys of the willingness of physicians and nurses to help in various types of disasters, which have found low levels for radiological incidents—45 to 57 percent (Lanzilotti et al., 2002; Qureshi et al., 2005);
- a belief that EDs and hospital facilities more generally are not sufficiently prepared for a terrorist event involving radioactive materials;
- lack of confidence about how to use detection equipment;

- lack of confidence that personal protective equipment (PPE) and hospital procedures will provide adequate protection from contamination of the hospital by patients; and
- personal safety in a chaotic situation.

There was also strong opposition from doctors and nurses participating in the study to a treatment protocol recommended by some agencies. Whereas in most cases patients are decontaminated first and then treated, in situations where an incoming patient has life-threatening injuries the protocol calls for treating and stabilizing the patient first and addressing decontamination issues afterward. The protocol is based on the idea that to delay treatment in such situations would result in patient deaths, and that the risk to health care workers would be minimal provided the patient's clothing is removed and standard radiation protection and ED practices are followed. A significant number of the physicians and nurses in the study, however, strongly rejected this idea, expressing the view that decontamination should always take place before any treatment is rendered.

Based on the full set of research studies noted above, Becker drew several overarching conclusions:

- An IND event will pose huge challenges in terms of emergency communication.
- Timely, effective messaging will be vital for reducing morbidity and mortality, preventing psychosocial and behavioral impacts, and maintaining public trust and confidence.
- Carrying out message research well in advance of any event is essential.
- Messages to the public need to focus strongly on health issues and concerns and involve spokespersons seen as credible on health issues.
- Emergency planners should recognize that willingness to shelter depends significantly on parents' confidence that their children in schools will be protected. This further emphasizes the importance of better linking school emergency planning to broader preparedness efforts.
- Fatalism among minority populations may need to be addressed through tailored or targeted messaging and other strategies.
- Unclear terms such as "shelter in place" need be replaced or explained more clearly.
- Emergency responders, while strongly committed to their professional duties, have deep concerns about radiation events and do not believe they or their organizations are adequately prepared. They are also concerned about the well-being of their families.

- Messages to and training of public health professionals need to better clarify public health's roles and responsibilities in radiological/nuclear incidents.
- There appears to be a difference between some official protocols and what hospital ED clinicians are actually willing to do in practice. This disjunction needs to be addressed.
- Health professionals have many deep concerns and uncertainties related to large-scale radiological emergencies. These need to be acknowledged and better addressed through training, communication, information, and other efforts.

H. Keith Florig presented the "mental models approach" to risk communication for lay decision making developed at Carnegie Mellon University (Morgan et al., 2002). The approach includes the following five steps:

1. Drawing on technical and decision experts to create a normative model of the recipients' decision
2. Using structured open-ended interviews to elicit laypersons' mental models of what the situation would be (e.g., "Tell me what you know about fallout")
3. Comparing expert and lay models to identify missing and erroneous concepts in expert and lay understanding of key issues (e.g., pieces of the expert model missing from the lay model, pieces of the lay model that are erroneous, and pieces in the lay model that do not exist in the expert model but that are still very important) (The importance that people put on the safety of their pets during Hurricane Katrina is a good example of something that the experts did not anticipate.)
4. Using the results to draft risk communication
5. Testing and refining communications with target populations to see what is still misinterpreted and to identify terms that are still ambiguous

The impetus for developing the mental-models approach to risk communication messaging was the realization that messages developed by subject-matter experts can fail to achieve their purpose because they are not designed to address recipients' decision needs (i.e., provide information relevant to the recipient's impending choices) and are not written in terms that the recipient can understand. Carnegie Mellon researchers have found through experience that the mental-models approach is best applied by an interdisciplinary team consisting of subject-matter specialists, decision analysts, behavioral scientists, and communication specialists.

The mental-models approach has not been used to develop risk communication strategies or message content specifically for a nuclear detonation event. Florig laid out how this might be done. He showed a normative model that he had developed of the decision to shelter or evacuate. He listed some questions that might be used to elicit lay peoples' mental models of the decision domain. Examples include, "Some people are worried that a terrorist group might be able to explode a nuclear weapon in a U.S. city. Can you tell me what people could do to protect themselves against such a possibility?" "You mentioned that the explosion would produce fallout. Can you elaborate?" These questions might discover that some people believe that fallout is only dangerous as the cloud goes over, or that they believe it will be dangerous for thousands of years. They might find that most people would try to escape in cars even though they were advised to shelter in place, because they did not understand the substantial shielding effect of buildings compared with cars.

After identifying missing or erroneous concepts of nuclear detonation hazards in the lay public, messages designed to counter them would be developed, then tested and refined. Currently, for example, DHS provides the following advice for responding to a nuclear blast:

1. Take cover immediately, below ground if possible, though any shield or shelter will help protect you from the immediate effects of the blast and the pressure wave.
2. Consider if you can get out of the area.
3. Or consider if it would be better to go inside a building and follow your plan to "shelter in place."[34]

This message could be tested in structured interviews with individuals or in focus groups. Such testing might find that the advice is not specific enough (it mentions getting out of the area without specifying what "the area" or "out of the area" would be), not complete enough (it does not mention children), or not clear enough (the meaning of the term "shelter in place" may not be evident to some people).

Next, Florig presented an analysis that a colleague and he had conducted of the value to an individual of preparing for sheltering (Florig and Fischhoff, 2007). They calculated the initial and annual maintenance costs of a stock of sheltering supplies specified in federal guidelines. The initial stocking cost of these supplies is estimated to be about $300, with continuing costs of about $250 per year to replace perishables (e.g., food and medicine) and to cover rent on the storage space. Such an expense may not be affordable for some people, and those who can afford it may choose not to invest in supplies if

---

[34] See http://www.ready.gov/america/_downloads/nuclear.pdf (accessed June 23, 2009).

they see too little chance of benefiting from the investment. If one assumes, for instance, that there is a 1 percent chance of a nuclear event in one's city over the next 10 years, the odds of shelter preparations actually saving a person's life would be only a few chances in 100,000.[35] To invest in shelter preparation under these conditions, one would have to have a willingness to pay for risk reduction of approximately $50 million per life saved. This far exceeds what people seem willing to pay for a unit of risk reduction in other personal contexts. Likewise, it is much greater than the value per statistical life measure recently used by DHS in evaluating regulations, which was $6.3 million in 2007 dollars (Robinson, 2008).

Ann Norwood focused on the psychological effects of an IND event in (1) the area hit by the immediate effects of the explosion, (2) area hospitals, and (3) the rest of the country. In the immediate area of the blast, one of the most important variables would be the speed with which people learned that it was a nuclear event and acted accordingly to avoid injury or further injury. Initially, there would be widespread shock and disbelief, confusion and disorientation, and fear. The urgency to reunite with loved ones would be intense and would possibly lead to additional exposure to dangerous levels of radiation. The sight of the dead and injured and the widespread destruction would cause horror. The disorientation caused by the horror would be reinforced by any deafness, blindness, brain trauma from the shockwave, or other injuries caused by the explosion.

Meanwhile, health care workers at hospitals would face an enormous influx of people looking for treatment or missing loved ones or seeking a save haven. There would be mass confusion and a lack of information about the nature and extent of the hazards caused by the explosion and the fallout. Workers could feel helpless due to overwhelming numbers of patients and rapidly depleted resources. Mass triage and treating patients under severely resource-constrained conditions would be psychologically difficult. Meanwhile, health care workers would be worried about the well-being of their own families and friends. In the long run, the traumatic experience of

---

[35] This figure was reached by assigning odds to a series of events leading to lethal exposure to fallout:

- Odds of an attack in my city: 0.2
- If attack happens in my city, wind will be blowing toward my house: 0.2
- If wind is blowing toward my house, I will be home: 0.3
- If I am at home, a timely alert will be issued: 0.5
- If alert is timely, I will hear it in time to take shelter: 0.5
- If I hear it, I will decide to shelter rather than flee: 0.5
- If I decide to shelter, my shelter will save me: 0.5
- Overall odds that shelter will save my life: 4 in 100,000

a mass casualty event would probably result in some health care workers being unable to keep working, as happened with emergency response personnel involved in the Oklahoma City Federal Building bombing.

Outside the immediate blast zone, there would be extensive fear of exposure to fallout and the desire of some people to be evaluated and treated, while others would be looking for a safe haven. As radiation levels fell, the number of patients from the fallout zone would increase. The demand for medical information would be high, not only about short-term consequences but also about long-term risk of cancer. Mothers with small children and pregnant women would be especially concerned about possible exposure and its effects.

In many people, fear and anxiety would result in self-protective behaviors and compliance with directions from authorities. In others, however, such fears would lead to apathy and inaction or, at the other extreme, panic and disorganization. High anxiety would have a variety of physiological effects, such as chest pain, diarrhea, dizziness, faintness, flushing (or pallor) of the skin, hyperventilation, nausea and vomiting, palpitations, and tachycardia. Some of these effects of anxiety mimic symptoms of ARS (e.g., nausea, vomiting, and diarrhea). In the Goiânia incident, for example, 11 percent of the 112,000 who showed up to be assessed for contamination exhibited nausea, reddened skin, and other potential symptoms of ARS. After they were found to be uncontaminated, the symptoms disappeared within several hours.[36]

The impact that an IND incident would have on the rest of the country is difficult to predict. Just-in-time education about radiation effects and hazards would probably be needed in areas receiving refugees of such an event. Residents of Goiânia, for example, were subject to discrimination when they traveled (e.g., not being allowed to board airplanes, being asked not to use swimming pools or other public facilities at hotels, and so forth) because of lack of understanding that the victims of whole-body radiation are not radioactive. More than 8,000 of the 112,000 residents who showed up for examination asked for an official certificate that they were not contaminated.

Norwood concluded with remarks about the difficulty of preparing for an IND event. In her view, the challenge is to increase the public's understanding of radiation and protective measures to take in the event of a nuclear detonation without scaring people unnecessarily.

Dori Reissman also addressed the extreme stress and psychological trauma likely to occur because of an IND detonation and the effects that follow. She focused on the impact that the confusion, disorientation, and

---

[36] Norwood cited Collins (2002) for this information.

fear caused by tremendous uncertainty, high stress, and psychosocial trauma would have on the quality of the decisions made by people and leaders about how to respond to the nuclear detonation. People would be wondering whether they were being exposed to radiation and where it was safe and where it was dangerous to be. They would be deciding whether to seek shelter immediately or to evacuate. Many would be deciding whether to find their children or other family members before sheltering or evacuating. They would be deciding whether to seek medical screening for exposure to radiation.

Stress would have adverse effects on decision making because the general public and leaders would likely have trouble concentrating and would find it harder to assimilate new information. Stress could cause a variety of symptoms that might make some people think they had been exposed to radiation. Massive numbers of people might seek medical care who do not really need it (something that happened following the radiation incident in Goiânia and the sarin gas attack in Tokyo).

According to the research literature, it is often the case that much of the public fails to adhere to recommended public health actions. After the 2001 anthrax attacks, for example, less than half (44 percent) of the individuals at high risk of anthrax exposure from the attacks completed the recommended course of antibiotics. A number of people refused to evacuate during Hurricane Katrina.

Poor compliance with public health recommendations may be attributed to messaging that is not complete or clear or consistent, lack of trust of public authorities, or the beliefs, prejudices, and misconceptions of the public. Complete and clear guidance is usually necessary but not sufficient to motivate appropriate behavior. Part of the solution is to establish trust in leadership; part of it is showing people that there are benefits that outweigh the risks if they behave according to recommendations.

Reissman stressed that leadership has a key role in establishing the trust necessary for people to accept information and guidance, especially if that information or guidance is counterintuitive. Should they, for instance, act on advice to evacuate or to shelter? Authorities should be perceived as caring, calm, and knowledgeable, which requires consistency in approaches to messaging.

The goal should be to create public trust and to shape behavior in such a way as to reduce risk, both among the public and among first responders and health care providers. Members of the latter groups will be concerned about the well-being of their families during the event. They also may be concerned about discrimination and stigma, especially concerning their children when they go back to school. This happened in the case of children of postal workers who worked at the facilities contaminated with anthrax in 2001. Some people shunned these children because they wrongly thought they were possibly contaminated with anthrax or, if infected, could infect others.

Discussion of Risk Communication, Public Reactions, and Psychological Consequences

A participant noted that, during the first Gulf War, DoD communicated the answers to the questions it thought were important very well, but failed to anticipate some of the soldiers' questions. For example, DoD was not prepared for questions about the genetic effects of chemical and radiological hazards on children the solders might have in the future. The participant suggested making an effort to understand what responders would be concerned about and having the information and advice ready in advance. Panelists agreed with this, concluding that if medical authorities did not deal with the public's questions, they would have trouble hearing what authorities wanted to tell them because people would place their concerns first.

There was discussion of the advisability of giving placebos—or KI pills, which would be harmless if they were not needed—to people who fear they have been exposed in order to ease their anxiety and stress. The panelists strongly opposed this because of professional ethics but also because it would undermine public trust in authorities, which would be critical to maintain in such a situation. Ursano, a committee member, noted that medications and non-medication-based therapies are currently under study to be given immediately for the prevention of psychiatric disease resulting from traumatic stress. It is possible, for example, that many cases of PTSD can be successfully treated. According to research studies, early initiation of cognitive behavioral therapy about 3 weeks after exposure to a traumatic event will substantially reduce the rates of PTSD. However, less is understood about the efficacy of public health interventions.

Florig clarified that the development of an expert model of what is important for the public to know and do is not aimed at establishing what public health authorities should motivate people to do. Rather, it is part of a process of comparing expert and public concepts of what is important in order to produce a convergence of message content that would be faithful to both scientific knowledge and to what people believe and value.

A workshop participant asked if there was an assessment instrument that could be used for the triage of mass psychological casualties in the field. Such instruments do exist. For example, PsySTART, a rapid mental health triage and incident management system developed for children, was mentioned (Schreiber, 2005). Rather than identifying symptoms, which can take time to appear, those instruments identify risk factors that may lead to patients developing psychiatric problems. There is emerging evidence that brief mental health interventions in the first few weeks after a traumatic event can reduce long-term morbidity.

The 12-item SPRINT-E (Short PTSD Rating Interview-Expanded Version) (Norris et al., 2008) and the 6- or 10-item Kessler Psychological

Distress Scale (Kessler et al., 2002), which are used to estimate the prevalence of mental illness in populations, were also mentioned. However, there are no standardized instruments in common use today.

A participant wondered how to communicate with the public about an issue on which there is no consensus among experts—for example, at what number of cGy units should treatment be started. Becker said that there are many examples of situations in which divided messages or conflicting signals are sent, and these never turn out well in terms of messaging or how well the population complies with the recommendations. Where consensus does not exist, he said that experts should try to develop it, especially on issues for which messages need to be prepared in advance. Florig urged input from the public, especially in situations for which blanket advice is not appropriate, such as what to do about fallout. He supported a model in which the goal is to provide people with the information they need to make a good decision for themselves, based on their particular situations. If scientific knowledge or consensus does not exist, people should be informed of this so that they can deal with the ambiguity. Reissman's view was that the technical community is needed to define what to do based on evidence, but the behavioral research community is also needed to help inform how best to help people cope with the uncertainties inherent in such events.

A participant involved in hospital preparedness affirmed that people do not always know what "shelter in place" means and suggested the following guidelines as being much more clear to people: "When something is really bad outside, you stay in, and when something is really bad inside, you go out."

There was a question about panic. Ursano responded that the literature on disasters shows that panic is a rare phenomenon. When it occurs, it is generally related to a lack of ability to leave or to concerns about children.

The treatment of contaminated patients was discussed. Daniel Flynn, a committee member, expressed concern that health care providers would not understand and thus would exaggerate the risks involved in treating an externally contaminated victim with serious physical trauma or burns, and therefore would want more decontamination than is necessary, or called for, by protocols. More patients would die than would be necessary in that situation. For example, a victim arriving at an ED might give off radiation at the rate of 25 millirem per hour. The Geiger counter would sound an ominous audio signal, but even if the patient were in surgery for 20 hours, the accumulated dose to the medical personnel would be half a rem (5 mSv) (about half the dose from one abdominal computerized tomography scan). However, with the removal of clothes and wiping down of exposed skin and hair, most of the contamination would be removed, reducing the absorbed dose to health care personnel to a few millirem or less (much less that a chest X-ray). Becker said his interviews with health care providers found little confidence that they would receive accurate information or a full picture of the situation, and they told him that they do not want to find out later that they have made a fatal error.

A participant suggested working on consistency among the DHS, HHS, and CDC websites. The agencies have significant differences in their standards, but efforts like Pandemicflu.com show that with work, the agencies could develop a single message.

SUMMARY OF KEY POINTS FROM THE JUNE WORKSHOP

Jerome Hauer was asked to sum up the main issues and points brought up during the June workshop. He began with the statement that at this time no city is prepared to handle the aftermath of an IND detonation. Few have even begun to make plans, although there is some progress on preparing for an RDD attack. One reason he identified was the expectation of local officials that the federal agencies would arrive, take over, and provide all the support needed in the aftermath. Also, because the federal agencies have not adequately communicated with local officials about what they would be dealing with, the local officials do not have all the information they need to begin realistic planning for such an eventuality.

Hauer asserted that the health care system in this country is totally unprepared to handle the surge in demand that will occur in the aftermath of an IND event. This is particularly true of beds for burn patients. There are plans to put beds in hallways, but with few exceptions the infrastructure for this (e.g., electrical outlets, oxygen sources, plumbing outlets in the halls) is not there.

There is also the problem of the probable loss of health care facilities, staff, and emergency responders that would result from a 10-kt explosion (e.g., police, fire, EMS, ED doctors and nurses, public health workers). Many of those who survive will be diverted by concerns about the safety of their families and about their own personal safety. Those who survive and report to work will be hampered by conflicting information about the effects of radiation dose rates and total accumulated doses on their health and about what to do about any exposure to radiation they may have received.

First responders need more training on responding to an IND incident. The existing planning and training for RDDs is further along, but an IND would be a very different scenario and would demand a very different response.

There is a lack of tools for estimating the radiation exposure levels of victims in the field beyond documenting time to vomiting, an imperfect measure. Even in hospitals, fecal and urine testing, lymphocyte kinetics and cytogenetics, and other procedures to assess the degree of exposure and to guide treatment might be available for incidents involving one or a few radiation victims but would not be practical in a mass casualty incident.

Preparedness for evacuation of people under the fallout plume is a "confusing mess." There is little capacity to communicate with the population about the situation and to provide them with advice and guidance in the event of an IND detonation. Consistency of message content is also lacking. On what basis will authorities advise people to leave the fallout area or to stay where they are? If the recommendation is to stay in place, how will people be supported if they need food or medical care or other basic services to last several days? These are also issues in planning for an influenza pandemic.

If people evacuate, what are the plans for maintaining them somewhere else? In addition to logistics, receiving communities may fear contamination from people who come from the vicinity of the nuclear detonation.

Consistent messaging is also needed for emergency responders on the criteria for entering the fallout area. When is it safe for them to conduct rescue operations, and how will they know? Even if radiation dropped rapidly to levels that would not cause acute injury, it would still be somewhat elevated and would increase cancer rates in the longer term. What information will first responders need to make decisions and how will this information get to them? More work needs to be done on developing and communicating consistent guidelines on acceptable exposure levels.

Consistent and useful messaging will also be critical in avoiding a loss of confidence in the government. Messages will need to go out immediately. If they are not consistent, they will reduce confidence in the government and will amplify rather than alleviate stress and fear. The media will need to be briefed as part of the preparedness for terrorist attacks with WMDs such as an IND, and they should be involved in exercises. Inconsistent messages from government officials and the media were a major problem in the response to the anthrax attacks in 2001.

Moving patients would be difficult because of concerns about radiation contamination among people in the receiving cities. Furthermore, cities not hit by an IND might be reluctant to fill their hospital beds with the injured from other cities until they are sure they are not going to be attacked themselves.

Much more training is needed for pre-hospital care providers and hospital medical staff about performing triage in a mass casualty situation. The training is especially needed for responding to a nuclear event because the degree of radiation exposure among victims will be difficult to determine, which in turn will make it difficult to separate those who do not need treatment from those who have received fatal doses or from those who could benefit from treatment.

A system for resupplying hospitals will be necessary, because currently they practice supply chain management and only store a day or two of drugs and other medical supplies.

Countermeasure development should be accelerated. No licensed countermeasures exist for the acute radiation injury that would result from an IND detonation. Currently licensed countermeasures hasten the excretion or block the effects of internalized radionuclides, but internal contamination would not be a major contributor to the acute morbidity and mortality produced by such an event.

Psychosocial effects can be expected to be substantial and will have to be handled at the local level. A capacity to mitigate the psychosocial impacts of the confusion and fear of an IND attack must be part of the preparedness effort, so that people will be able to make better decisions about protecting themselves during the event and will not develop long-term mental depression, PTSD, or other anxiety disorders.

Finally, the threat of terrorist INDs should be better communicated to state and local officials and responders. Currently, they have their plates full with preparedness for chemical attacks, RDDs, and other immediate concerns. INDs seem on the one hand to be a remote threat and on the other to be too overwhelming and too catastrophic for which to try to prepare. The impossibility of preparing for nuclear events may have been true during the Cold War, when the scenarios of concern entailed the simultaneous detonation of hundreds or thousands of warheads, but the terrorist IND threat is comparatively limited in scope and improved preparedness to respond could save thousands of lives.

TOPIC 6: FEDERAL AND STATE MEDICAL RESOURCES FOR RESPONDING TO AN IND EVENT

Judith Monroe, the committee member moderating this August workshop panel, opened by citing two recent examples of public health emergencies that took place in Indiana—a full-scale exercise run by the Indiana National Guard (2007) and an actual event, the emergency evacuation of a hospital in Indiana due to flooding (2008).

The 2007 Ardent Sentry exercise in Indiana was conducted to test the military's ability to collaborate with nonmilitary emergency responders in responding to a domestic incident of national significance. The scenario was an IND detonation in Indianapolis, tainting the water, destroying seven hospitals, and putting 300,000 people on the roads trying to escape. It was a several-day exercise involving about 5,000 participants, including hundreds of simulated casualties. The exercise revealed communication and coordination problems stemming from the mismatch between the military's top-down organization and the civilian bottom-up structure. Also, emergency responders found it difficult to develop a common operating picture or implement a common plan, which led Indiana to increase training in these skills. Communication problems led to a delayed activation of the National Disaster Medical System (NDMS).

The 2008 incident in Indiana was an actual public health emergency. Flooding forced the evacuation of a 135-bed hospital, 2 nursing homes, a dialysis clinic, and 8 group homes near Columbus. The hospital basement was flooded, destroying the power generators and the laboratory, and all entrances but one were blocked. The hospital staff learned that there was no time to pull their plans from the shelf and that, in any case, the plans did not fit the circumstances. They found instead that they benefited greatly from a functional exercise that they had conducted a year earlier. Although the exercise was for a mass casualty surge situation rather than an evacuation, the prior experience with the Incident Command System was very valuable. The Indiana National Guard, whose base was nearby, assisted in the evacuation and provided security. The Carolinas MED-1 unit with its mobile hospital was brought in to provide services while the flooded hospital was out of commission.

Monroe introduced the panel, which consisted of U.S. Public Health Service Captain Ann Knebel, deputy director of preparedness planning in the Office of the Assistant Secretary for Preparedness and Response (ASPR) at HHS; Alan Remick, consequence management program coordinator in the Office of Emergency Response of the National Nuclear Security Administration at DOE; Col. Daniel Bochicchio of the National Defense University and, until recently, vice chief surgeon in the National Guard Bureau; and James Blumenstock, who is with the Association of State and Territorial Health Officials.

Ann Knebel began by providing an overview of the medical assets that HHS could deploy in a nuclear event as well as of HHS's response plans. HHS has a number of medical assets, and she described the major ones among them:

- *Medical Reserve Corps (MRC).* MRC is composed of more than 160,000 medical and public health professionals organized in approximately 700 units across the country who serve as volunteers in responses to natural disasters and emergencies.
- *Emergency System for Advance Registration of Volunteer Health Professionals (ESAR-VHP).* ESAR-VHP is composed of individual health professionals who volunteer to help in emergencies.

- *National Disaster Medical System (NDMS)*. NDMS is a cooperative effort of HHS, DHS, DoD, and the Department of Veterans Affairs (VA) to supplement state and local medical resources during major disasters or emergencies.[37]

  NDMS has three components: (1) approximately 5,000 volunteers in 93 response teams, most of them disaster medical assistance teams (DMATs) for general disaster medical assistance, but some specializing in areas such as burns, pediatrics, and mental health; (2) approximately 1,800 nonfederal hospitals that have volunteered to provide approximately 110,000 acute care beds in a national emergency, along with VA hospitals; and (3) aeromedical evacuation services provided by DoD using Air Force assets and, if needed, the Civil Reserve Air Fleet (CRAF).

  A fully operational, or Level One, DMAT response team has 35 medical and paramedical members, is ready to deploy in 6 hours, can be on the ground and operational within 48 hours, and is equipped to treat 250 ambulatory patients a day (or 125 patients a day including approximately 8 inpatients at a time and limited laboratory and pharmacy services) for 3 days without resupply. A National Medical Response Team with 50 members is trained to provide medical care following a nuclear, biological, or chemical incident, including mass casualty decontamination, medical triage, and primary and secondary medical care to stabilize victims for transportation to tertiary care facilities in a hazardous material environment.

- *U.S. Public Health Service commissioned corps teams*. There are five rapid deployment force (RDF) teams, one of which is on 12-hour notice at any given time. Each RDF team has 105 officers with clinical, public health, or mental health expertise.

- *Radiation Event Medical Management (REMM)*. REMM is an online tool developed by ASPR and the National Library of Medicine. REMM can be accessed for just-in-time information and treatment protocols for radiation exposure (Bader et al., 2008).

- *Radiation Injury Treatment Network (RITN)*. RITN was established by ASPR, the National Marrow Donor Program, and the National Cancer Institute. It is composed of transplant and cancer centers familiar with treating bone marrow suppression and other aspects of radiation injury (Weinstock et al., 2008).

- *Radiation Treatment, Triage, and Transport (RTR) system*. The RTR system is being developed by HHS as a model for medical response to a nuclear detonation. The concept is to collect victims

---

[37] NDMS also provides backup medical support to the military and VA medical care systems during an overseas conventional conflict.

in three types of locations by type of medical problem: (1) those with major trauma who were in the high radiation zone around ground zero, (2) those without traumatic injury but at high risk of developing ARS, and (3) those with minimal or no radiation exposure and no significant trauma who do not require immediate medical care. Victims would then be directed to medical care sites, if they need immediate medical care, or assembly centers, if they do not need immediate medical care (Coleman et al., 2008; Vanderwagen, 2008).[38]

Under the NRF, HHS is the lead federal agency for public health and medical services in a national emergency. In this role HHS coordinates the activities of the other federal agencies with relevant assets and programs under Emergency Support Function #8 (ESF-8), "Public Health and Medical Services." HHS also has a broad public health and medical services role under the Nuclear/Radiological Incident Annex to the NRF.[39]

ASPR, under the broad guidelines of the NRF and related policy documents, such as ESF-8 and the NRF nuclear/radiological annex, has been developing "playbooks" for each of the 15 NRF National Planning Scenarios, including Scenario 1, which is the detonation of a 10-kt IND. Each playbook includes sections on the scenario, a concept of operations (CONOPS) for the response, action steps, pre-scripted mission subtasks, and essential elements of information. CONOPS specifies the role of each agency, and the action steps include a trigger for each step, a recommended strategy to follow, and specific actions to take. ASPR has put the playbooks for hurricanes and aerosolized anthrax attacks on its website so that state and local planners can see what federal capabilities might be deployed and how.[40] ASPR plans to publish each of the playbooks, with the ones for RDD and pandemic influenza events as the next to be posted.[41]

Alan Remick summarized DOE's resources for responding to a nuclear event such as a terrorist IND attack. The mission of DOE's Office of Emergency Response in the National Nuclear Security Administration is to provide expert technical information and advice in a nuclear radiological event.

---

[38] After the workshop, more details about RTR were released (EOP, 2009:65-67).

[39] The NRF, Nuclear/Radiological Incident Annex to the NRF, and ESF-8 can be found at http://www.fema.gov/emergency/nrf/ (accessed June 23, 2009).

[40] The playbooks are at http://www.hhs.gov/disasters/discussion/planners/Playbook/ (accessed June 23, 2009).

[41] As of June 29, 2009, the pandemic influenza playbook had been added to the ASPR website and the RDD playbook was indicated as "coming soon" (http://www.hhs.gov/disasters/discussion/planners/playbook/).

Specifically, DOE has a number of rapidly deployable capabilities that it can use in responding to a broad range of radiological incidents, such as those involving nuclear power or nuclear weapons production facilities, a nuclear weapons accident, or lost or stolen radioactive materials.[42] The capabilities most relevant to consequence management in response to a large-scale radiation event such as the detonation of an IND include the following:

- *Atmospheric Release Advisory Capability (ARAC)*. ARAC, located at Lawrence Livermore National Laboratory, has sophisticated computer models that can provide near-real-time assessments of the consequences of actual or potential radiation releases by modeling the movement of hazardous plumes. The plume models are based on real-time weather data, a terrain database, and a three-dimensional transport and diffusion model. The model results are presented in terms of ground deposition plots, instantaneous and time-integrated doses, and airborne concentrations, which can be used to inform protective action decisions. ARAC is available 24 hours a day.

- *Aerial Measuring System (AMS)*. AMS has aviation-based equipment capable of surveying large areas in response to radiological emergencies. An all-weather fixed-wing aircraft can arrive quickly to perform quick radiation surveys of an area where fallout has been deposited and where exposure rates are very high. Helicopters arrive more slowly but can conduct detailed aerial surveys over the course of several days and produce exposure-rate contour maps and determine which isotopes are involved.

- *Radiological Assistance Program (RAP)*. Seven-person RAP teams are based around the country, with at least three in each of nine regions (with most team members working in one of the national laboratories). The teams would arrive within 6 hours of an event to assist state, local, and other federal agencies in the detection, identification, and analysis of radioactive materials (such as fallout) and with the appropriate response to an event involving radiological or nuclear material. The teams' expertise includes assessment, area

---

[42] These include, for example, the Nuclear/Radiological Advisory Team (NRAT), which provides advice and limited technical assistance (e.g., search, diagnostics, effects prediction) as part of a Domestic Emergency Support Team; Search Response Teams (SRTs), which, using local support, engage in initial nuclear search activities; and the Accident Response Group, which provides technical response to U.S. nuclear weapons accidents. The purpose of NRAT and SRT is detection and interdiction of a nuclear release before it happens, and they were not discussed at the workshop, although presumably they would be searching for possible additional INDs if one were detonated somewhere in the United States.

monitoring, air sampling, and exposure and contamination control. They would be a resource for the local incident commander.

- *Radiation Emergency Assistance Center/Training Site (REAC/TS).* Located at Oak Ridge, Tennessee, REAC/TS is staffed with physicians and health physicists who conduct training on the medical aspects of radiation exposure and who are available at all times to deploy and provide EMS at radiation incidents. In the event of an IND detonation, REAC/TS is not large enough to deploy and treat people, but it would provide advice and consultation on radiation emergency medicine. It has one of the few U.S. cytogenetic dosimetry laboratories, but these laboratories would be quickly overwhelmed in a mass casualty nuclear situation. It has a stockpile of DTPA and Prussian Blue, but the stockpile is very small compared with the amounts in the SNS. Perhaps its main contribution in the immediate response to an IND detonation would be the state and local responders it has trained in emergency radiation medicine, some of whom would likely be onsite or nearby.
- *Federal Radiological Monitoring and Assessment Center (FRMAC).* FRMAC would integrate the various DOE assets to provide a common operating picture of the radiological environment for whoever is managing the incident. FRMAC is a multiagency organization that would also include response personnel from EPA, DoD, National Guard, and other agencies.

Ideally, the DOE response would take place according to the following pattern:

- ARAC would provide an initial predictive plot of the plume based on actual weather conditions and what is known about the location and size of the explosion within 15 minutes and then update the plot as information about the actual deposition and radiation levels was received.
- An AMS aircraft would be dispatched immediately from Nellis or Andrews Air Force Base and begin transmitting rough radiation survey data soon after arrival.
- RAP teams would be dispatched from the nearest region or regions within a few hours and begin arriving within 12 hours.

The FRMAC response would be phased:

- A Consequence Management Home Team, physically based at Nellis Air Force Base in Las Vegas, Nevada, would gather available data within 2 hours and provide whatever information it could to the incident command.

- A Phase 1 Consequence Management Response Team (CMRT) of 26 people would leave Nellis Air Force Base within 4 hours and be on site within 6-10 hours with some equipment to establish the FRMAC and conduct some gross field monitoring and data assessment in order to understand better the locations of the radiation and fallout.
- A Phase 2 CMRT with much more equipment and supplies (15 tons) would arrive within 24 hours and begin more extensive field monitoring and sampling of air, water, and ground concentrations of radiation; map the actual path of the fallout plume; and provide exposure-rate and dose-projection contour maps for officials managing the response.
- A full interagency FRMAC would be operational within 24 to 36 hours and consist of up to 500 people as the situation warranted, which an IND incident surely would. Eventually, when the situation had stabilized and attention turned to recovery and clean-up, EPA would take over FRMAC from DOE.

In summary, DOE would send specialized personnel and equipment to determine where and how much radiation was produced by an IND detonation, provide this information and expert advice to those managing the response, and through REAC/TS provide expert advice on medical matters. The total number of DOE people involved in the emergency response would be approximately 1,200.

Daniel Bochicchio reviewed the assets and expected role of the National Guard in an IND event. The Army National Guard has about 355,000 members and the Air National Guard has approximately another 106,000. More than half of them are available for domestic emergencies at any given time, while one quarter are deployed in Iraq and Afghanistan and another quarter are preparing for deployment.

National Guard medical capabilities include the following:

- Medical triage
- Emergency medical treatment
- Patient evacuation
- Preventive medicine and critical incident stress management teams
- Limited hospitalization

The National Guard has

- seven multifunctional medical battalion command and control headquarters (one of which is deployed overseas);
- sixteen air ambulance companies (five of which are deployed or getting ready to deploy). Each air ambulance company has 12 helicopters capable of short-range medical evacuation;
- six ground ambulance companies, each with 24 ambulances;
- twenty-two area support medical companies, each with eight ambulances, able to provide emergency medical treatment (six companies are deployed or are getting ready to deploy);
- twenty-eight brigade support medical companies, each with eight ambulances, able to provide emergency medical treatment (six companies are deployed or are getting ready to deploy). These companies are part of a combat brigade and would deploy with their brigade if it were called on to respond to an IND event;
- nine Expeditionary Medical Support+25 (EMEDS+25) rapid response packages in Washington State, Kansas, and Pennsylvania, which can be transported in a C-130 (an EMEDS+25 cares for a population at risk of 2,000-5,000 with 9 tents, an Air National Guard Medical Service staff of 85, 25 critical care beds, and laboratory, radiology, pharmacy, and dental ancillary services. The purpose of EMEDS is to provide initial surge capacity while other facilities are being ramped up); and
- ten aeromedical evacuation squadrons, each with a mobile staging facility able to prepare about 40 patients an hour for aeromedical transport.

In addition,

- Each state has a WMD Civil Support Team (CST).[43] Each CST consists of 22 people (4 of them medical and 8 emergency responders), a command vehicle, an operations van, a communications vehicle, and an analytical laboratory van to test environmental samples. CSTs are on constant standby and can deploy an advance party within 90 minutes and the rest of the team within 3 hours. The CST commander advises the civilian incident commander on the type and level of chemical, biological, radiological, nuclear, or explosive (CBRNE) hazard; current and projected consequences;

---

[43] There are 55 total. California has two. The District of Columbia, Guam, Puerto Rico, and the U.S. Virgin Islands also have teams.

possible response measures; and availability of additional National Guard assets.

- Seventeen states have a CBRNE Enhanced Response Force Package (CERFP). Each CERFP has four elements: search and extraction, decontamination, medical, and command and control. The medical element consists of 30 to 45 physicians, physician assistants, nurses, and medics from the Air National Guard Medical Service.

CSTs are intended to augment local first responders by assessing and identifying CBRNE threats. CERFPs are intended to provide extraction, decontamination, and medical triage and treatment in the period from 6 hours post-incident to the time when substantial National Guard and military forces arrive 72 to 96 hours after detonation. These capabilities would be relatively small, however, relative to the needs generated by an IND event, with 22 and up to approximately 200 personnel, respectively. Barring additional incidents, however, a state's CST and CERFP could be supplemented by those of nearby states under the Emergency Management Assistance Compact (EMAC).[44]

James Blumenstock reviewed the preparedness of the state and territorial public health departments—especially the five states containing the six Tier 1 UASI cities—for the medical consequences of an IND detonation. The state health departments would adhere to the NRF, its Nuclear/Radiological Incident Annex, and ESF-8, and they are cognizant of National Planning Scenario 1, "Nuclear Detonation—10-Kiloton Improvised Nuclear Device" (as well as Scenario 11, "Radiological Attack—Radiological Dispersal Devices").

The states are engaged in all-hazards emergency preparedness, which does not necessarily guarantee that they will be prepared for every incident-specific issue associated with an IND or any other specific threat. Blumenstock emphasized that the states do not know the relative threat posed by INDs and that the 15 National Planning Scenarios are not ranked by importance. There is growing awareness of the possibility of and some planning for RDD attacks, but many states are generally just beginning to consider preparedness for an IND detonation. Currently, state public health

---

[44] After the workshop, NORTHCOM (United States Northern Command), DoD's command and control organization responsible for responding to terrorist attacks on the United States, established the first of three Chemical, Biological, Nuclear, or Radiation Consequence Management Response Task Forces. The 4,700-person task forces will have three units, whose jobs are to (1) conduct assessment and reconnaissance of an event to determine what agent or element is involved and to perform some emergency medical evacuations; (2) provide more significant medical assistance, patient decontamination, and evacuation; and (3) provide logistical support (Kreisher, 2008).

departments are most focused on preparedness for anthrax attacks and for an influenza pandemic, as well as for hurricanes, earthquakes, and other traditional natural hazards.

The priority given to anthrax and pandemic preparedness has been reflected in federal funding programs. The largest source of federal funding for public health preparedness, CDC's Public Health Emergency Preparedness (PHEP) grant program, provided approximately $5.5 billion in grants to states and localities between fiscal year (FY) 1999 and FY 2008 plus another $765 million in categorical grants in recent years. Most of the categorical grant funding has been specifically for pandemic influenza preparedness ($424 million) and preparedness for an anthrax attack through the CRI ($243 million).

Although in FY 2008 the PHEP program no longer included categorical grants for pandemic influenza, continued eligibility is tied to having an acceptable operations plan to address it based on guidance provided by HHS. There has been no PHEP funding specifically for radiological or nuclear event preparedness, although states (and localities) could allocate funds for them—or any other threat—from their basic PHEP funding, if it was a local priority. Similarly, the second largest source of funding for emergency preparedness, ASPR's Hospital Preparedness Program (HPP), does not make radiological or nuclear preparedness a priority. In fact, until FY 2008 HPP was the National Bioterrorism HPP.

State public health departments have competing priorities and they do not have the funding or staffing to deal with all of them. Furthermore, federal assistance for preparedness has been declining. PHEP funding fell by 30 percent from its high in FY 2002 to FY 2008, HPP funding fell by 20 percent from its high in FY 2004 to FY 2008, and the administration has again requested less funding for both programs for FY 2009.

Blumenstock did not advocate earmarking funding in PHEP or HPP for preparedness for an IND or any other specific threat; he made the point that other potential threats have been seen as relatively higher priority by the federal as well as the state governments.

Blumenstock stated that an IND detonation in a major metropolitan area would pose some incident-specific challenges:

- The effects would be catastrophic. Hundreds of thousands of people would be casualties and more than a million would be displaced by lingering radiation.
- There would be little to no warning before detonation.
- Local response capacity would be overwhelmed immediately.
- Local infrastructure would be destroyed.
- Federal assets would be needed and requested immediately.
- There would be unique long-term recovery and reentry issues.

The states with Tier 1 UASI cities contain among them approximately 35 nuclear power reactors, about a third of the nation's total, which they monitor and for which they prepare emergency response plans in case there is an accidental release of radiation. This gives them a head start on preparing for an IND detonation. They also have strengthened their all-hazards response capacity, most of which would be relevant in an IND incident. Regarding an IND event, Blumenstock says these states have begun to move beyond awareness to building more specific operational capacity and capability, and they have moved beyond the planning-to-plan stage to developing tangible plans. They are revising radiological response plans to include possible IND events. They are acquiring radiation detection and dosimetry equipment and modest stockpiles of radiation countermeasures and PPE. There is an effort to establish an East Regional Burn Consortium of health care facilities in the Mid-Atlantic and New England.

Blumenstock offered several recommendations to advance public health preparedness for the consequences of an IND event.

- Clarify the seriousness of the IND threat relative to current priorities (e.g., pandemic influenza and anthrax preparedness).
- Provide adequate funding, including federal, for preparedness.
- Improve federal coordination and find a federal agency leader or champion of IND event preparedness.
- Enhance the transfer of military knowledge, procedures, and experiential learning to the civilian public health sector.
- Improve medical countermeasures and related technologies.
- Strengthen the NDMS program to provide mass casualty care in the event of an IND detonation.

Discussion of Federal and State Medical Resources for Responding to an IND Event

The first topic was the level of interest on the part of states in developing their own pharmaceutical stockpiles for an IND event and the barriers they would face. Blumenstock said that there is interest and that the principal limiting factor is the lack of funding for acquiring and storing the stockpile. Furthermore, because the pharmaceuticals have a limited shelf life, state public health departments would be asking state legislators to commit to replacing the stockpile every 3 to 5 years with funding that could be used for more immediate needs, such as medical and social services.

A participant who works with state and local health departments said that, from his experience, few local emergency response managers in major U.S. cities know what federal assets would be available from the federal government. Moreover, there does not seem to be a point of contact at the federal level to determine what array of federal assets—civilian, National Guard, and military—would be brought to bear in particular kinds of emergencies. Knebel acknowledged that this is a problem, but she said that there has been incremental progress, citing the interagency process involved in developing the nuclear detonation playbook as a step toward providing the kind of transparency the participant wanted to see.[45] Additionally, there are 35 emergency coordinators stationed in the 10 Federal Emergency Management Agency (FEMA) regions who routinely engage in state-based exercises so that state and local officials understand what assets the federal government could provide in a public health and medical emergency. Federal funds are provided to support exercises that bring people together in order to discover gaps in preparedness. She noted that part of the problem is the high rate of turnover in state and local government personnel. Bochicchio said it was disappointing to find that the National Guard is not mentioned in some state pandemic influenza plans. On the other hand, in about 15 states, the adjutant general of the state's National Guard is also the state's emergency manager.

A participant with military experience said that for many years DoD planning focused on preventing nuclear events because to survive a Cold War nuclear exchange was considered impossible. Another scenario for which planning took place was a nuclear reactor accident. The current scenario is totally different. If an IND were used, survival would be considered feasible, but the consequences would be far more serious than a nuclear reactor accident. The infrastructure destruction would make it much more difficult to respond quickly and effectively. As seen in Hiroshima and Nagasaki, many people would have to rely on their own resources and response efforts. The participant pointed to the need for a massive public awareness campaign, perhaps similar to the duck-and-cover campaign of the 1950s.

Other participants doubted that people are ready to hear that the best way to defend themselves would be to stock up a shelter in a basement. Most people are not as concerned about such a low-probability event, despite the drastic consequences, as they are about an influenza pandemic or anthrax attack.

A participant suggested placing federal liaison officials in each major city in order to improve communication. ASPR has been reaching out with meetings in the states to build awareness of federal assets but it does not have funding for local liaison officers. A response was that appointing liaison officers in the six Tier 1 cities might be affordable.

A local public health preparedness official said he was aware that HHS and DOE have developed playbooks but that they have not been widely shared with the locals. He expressed a strong interest in sitting down with

---

[45] As noted in footnote 41, the IND playbook has not been released publicly.

federal partners and looking at their playbooks ahead of time. This would be important because, for example, when federal officials attending a recent state meeting on catastrophic earthquake planning said where they planned to establish collection points and landing sites for aeromedical evacuations, they discovered that there were major conflicts with that state's evacuation plans. State and local planners are determining where to put alternate care sites, points of pharmaceutical distribution, and other emergency arrangements, and broader plans up the line should be in harmony with the local plans. Or local plans might need to be adjusted to take advantage of federal plans and assets. Knebel said this was the purpose of posting the two (so far) playbooks online—so that local planners would know what HHS is planning.

A state emergency official said that one of the disconnects occurs when federal program officials bypass the state in dealing directly with localities, which creates confusion and conflict.

Bochicchio offered the military's practice of nesting plans, in which the tactical (i.e., local) plan or plans are nested within the operational (i.e., state or regional) plan, and the operational plan or plans are nested within the strategic (i.e., national) plan. What is not wanted, he said, is national planners conducting local tactical planning, which might not meet local reality or needs.

TOPIC 7: CURRENT PREPAREDNESS FOR RESPONDING TO THE IMMEDIATE CASUALTIES OF AN IND EVENT

George Annas, the committee member moderating the August workshop sessions related to Topic 7, began by noting that the IND detonation scenario in preparedness planning had raised at least six observations or questions regarding its usefulness:

1. Is the inability to quantify the risk, and the question of whether simply asserting it is "greater than zero," sufficient to motivate planners?
2. The general perception of planners is that the risk is so low or the response so inadequate that when first responders attend lectures on the topic their "eyes glaze over" and speakers are met with a "big yawn."
3. The "all-hazards" preparedness doctrine actually takes little or no account of the IND detonation scenario because of its unique characteristics.
4. A "worst-case scenario" can always be made worse.

5. Prevention is always preferable to reaction—which is especially true with nuclear scenarios.
6. It can, nonetheless, be useful to planners to use extreme situations, such as the IND detonation scenario, to test preparedness in general.

He then highlighted the major points from Hauer's summary of the June session of the workshop (presented earlier in this report):

- No city is prepared for, and few are focusing on, an IND event.
- Expectations are not well communicated among localities, states, and the federal government.
- The health care system is unprepared for a surge of patients, especially of burn victims.
- First responders need more training and direction in dealing with radiation and in triaging victims.
- The evacuation issue is central but unresolved at every level and will require good communication from and confidence in government.

Annas reviewed the format for the day, which consisted of short presentations from people involved in emergency medical responses in the Tier 1 UASI cities. The presentations under Topic 7 were organized into four panels, each of which addressed one of four questions about preparedness for the medical consequences of the immediate effects of an IND detonation. The four questions were as follows:

1. What is the capability to safely reach, triage, and perform prehospital treatment of those injured by the detonation? Would emergency responders be able to perform their duties in and around high-radiation areas?
2. What is the capacity to transport casualties to area treatment facilities? If emergency responders were able to reach, triage, and treat the injured, would they be able to evacuate and transport them to emergency care?
3. How prepared is the metropolitan area's medical system to treat casualties? Would health care facilities in the vicinity be able to handle the surge?
4. What is the preparedness to evacuate serious casualties to appropriate treatment facilities statewide and nationally? How would a large number of patients who need intensive treatment or supportive care for burns, trauma, or ARS be distributed among the limited number of intensive care units (ICUs) and burn beds in the nation?

Annas noted that the purpose of the presentations was not to evaluate the preparedness of any specific city or metropolitan area for an IND event. In fact, it was evident from the June session that no city is well prepared for an event with tens of thousands to hundreds of thousands of casualties and that the scale of resources needed to fill the gap is substantial. In addition, each city was represented by only approximately three officials, one each from the emergency medical response community, the local public health department, and the state public health department, which was not enough to evaluate any single city. Instead, the approach of the IOM committee was to assemble a pool of local and state officials actively involved in day-to-day emergency preparedness and response in order to obtain the local and state perspective on the major problems that they face—and the obstacles to solving them—in preparing for a catastrophic nuclear incident.

Panel 1 on Capability to Reach, Triage, and Treat the Injured

The presenters on this panel were John Brown from the San Francisco EMS Agency; Brooke Buddemeier from Lawrence Livermore National Laboratory; Michael Fitton from the Fire Department of New York; Kathleen "Cass" Kaufman from the Los Angeles County Department of Public Health; Joseph Newton from the Chicago Fire Department; and Richard Zuley from the Chicago Department of Public Health. They described their current efforts to prepare first responders for radiation and mass casualty incidents. At this point, most of the efforts to improve emergency response since 9/11 have been all-hazards in nature and not radiation-specific. The cities have been preparing for RDD events but are in the very early stages of preparing for an IND attack.

All-Hazards Preparedness

The Tier 1 UASI cities are training for and performing exercises with the Incident Command System, which is designed to coordinate the efforts of multiple agencies in a disaster. Still, it will be challenging to establish a unified command where everyone is working together in the case of an IND event. Not every locality has conducted a full-scale functional exercise that involves its entire system.

The Tier 1 UASI cities are improving their communication systems, especially in the area of interoperability of radios among fire and police and other first responders. Some now have hardened command centers. Not all radios are EMP-hardened, however.

There has been much training and upgrading of the credentials of first responders by, for example, training everyone in EMS—or everyone in the fire department, not just EMS personnel—in hazardous materials (hazmat) operations.

Cities have been developing agreements with their "collar" (surrounding) communities for assistance if they become overwhelmed. These agreements include EMS. There are agreements with private ambulance services to provide help, and there are arrangements with transit agencies to provide alternative means of transportation. These alternative means of transportation, which can include converted buses, mass transit vehicles, and ferries, are practiced at various mass events.

The cities have established alternative triage and collection points in such places as playgrounds and parks. There are also alternative aeromedical access sites.

Since major medical facilities, including Level 1 trauma centers, are often concentrated in the downtown area of a metropolitan area's central city, they may be unable to function in a major disaster such as an earthquake or hurricane, or following the detonation of an IND. Cities have been working on systems that can direct EMS to operational facilities.

Radiological Preparedness

Currently, the major cities are focusing on preparing for radiological emergencies, such as an RDD attack. First responders are being equipped with radiation detectors so that they can determine the level of radioactivity in their area and the level of a victim's contamination, and with personal dosimeters, so they would know the accumulated dose to which they have been exposed. Some even have equipment to identify the isotopes involved. They are being equipped with better PPE for CBRNE hazards, although PPE would protect a first responder only from contamination, not from penetrating external radiation, which would be the much greater hazard near ground zero.

First responders are trained and equipped to establish a perimeter around the radioactive zone surrounding the detonation point and to operate within that zone to save lives, perform prehospital care, and follow the hazmat decontamination process. Staffing cycles would be established to minimize exposure, and anyone reaching a PAG decision point, such as 50 rem for lifesaving activities, would be assigned to duty in nonradioactive zones.

IND Detonation Preparedness

There was clear recognition among the city representatives that the detonation of an IND would be at least an order of magnitude more disastrous than an RDD and that at least some of their health care facilities and personnel would be directly affected by the attack and thus unable to contribute to the response. Thus, the presenters spoke of the importance of regional arrangements with nearby jurisdictions, and with other states through the EMAC mechanism, to assist in the response. In addition, there was agreement that these mutual assistance arrangements must be exercised in advance, rather than being implemented for the first time during the event.

Generally, however, preparing specifically for a response to an IND detonation is in its early stages in most cities. Until recently, where WMDs in general are concerned, first responders have been concentrating primarily on preparedness for chemical and biological attacks; and where radiation threats are concerned, they have been paying more attention, as mentioned above, to planning a response to a radiological rather than a nuclear event.

One area of concern is the development of appropriate PAGs for responding to a nuclear detonation. To address these concerns, at least one jurisdiction is considering a higher decision point for first responders conducting lifesaving than the 50 rem (500 mSv) adopted for RDD and other radiological events. Currently, DHS's PAGs for RDD/IND do not have an upper limit, but they do set 25 rem (250 mSv) as the point beyond which a first responder must volunteer for lifesaving, must be informed of the possible acute and long-term effects of the exposure, and must be supplied with proper PPE. This follows the long-established EPA PAGs, which were developed for nuclear power plant accidents and lesser events (see previous section of this report). This lack of consensus at the local level reflects the lack of consensus at the federal level on the appropriate PAG decision point for working in the area immediately adjacent to an IND detonation point. (This issue is being worked on currently by a federal interagency group.)[46]

Related to this issue is the problem of knowing the location of the radioactive zones. At least some of the cities plan to tap into the federal sources of plume models and other information for the incident commander.

Yet another issue is whether and how to alter pre-hospital triage and treatment guidelines during a mass casualty event. The San Francisco EMS Agency has developed a mass casualty incident field operations guide that calls for the use of START or JumpSTART, followed by reevaluation of immediate and delayed patients for transport to a trauma center or specialty care, such as burn care. The agency also has a protocol for "austere" care during special circumstances (e.g., during a disaster when medical supplies are insufficient). This protocol, which must be authorized by the county health officer, is designed to provide a certain level of care to every individual who needs it instead of providing a high level of care to only a few individuals when emergency care resources are not adequate to provide

---

[46] The interagency group issued a report January 2009. See footnote 16 for a summary.

normal emergency care for everyone. There are also San Francisco Metropolitan Medical Response System (MMRS) medical treatment protocols for WMD incidents that apply at both the pre-hospital and hospital levels. In an IND event, both sets of protocols would be applied in conjunction with the triage guidelines for mass casualty incidents. The MMRS treatment protocols include protocols for radiation and blast injuries. Only advanced life support personnel would be allowed to enter a radioactive zone, which is where decontamination would be performed, and these personnel must consult a radiation safety officer if the projected dose is more than 5 rad.

At least one city has developed a training and information relationship with REAC/TS.

Even with well-conceived plans, the number of first responders would be small relative to the tens or hundreds of thousands of people injured by the immediate effects of an IND detonation. The Fire Department of the City of New York, for example, has only 35 HazTac and 5 paramedic rescue units in total that can work in radioactive zones. Overall, New York City's fire department ambulances average about 3,700 runs a day; Chicago's, by comparison, average about 900. San Francisco has between 12 and 24 ambulances in service, depending on the time of day, but could draw on as many as 70 private ambulances, each with a disaster kit sufficient to treat 50 victims and interoperable communications. It is clear that, even in our largest cities, the available resources, even assuming they remained fully operational, would be completely overwhelmed.

Discussion After Panel 1

A state EMS physician pointed out that all individuals working in the "hot zone" of high radioactivity around and immediately downwind of the detonation point will need active reading dosimeters so they will be able to monitor the total doses they have received. Some of the larger cities are acquiring these dosimeters, but most EMS systems do not have them.

There was a discussion of the difficulty of practicing large-scale EMS responses with suburban jurisdictions. No one wants to put 20 ambulances out of service for training. To help ambulances from other jurisdictions in mutual aid events, Chicago has set up four access points where ambulances coming from outside the city can pick up global positioning system (GPS) locators containing an automatic mapping system with the capabilities of different hospitals and providers. Houston also has established a staging area for mutual aid partners to pick up radios and be assigned a communication channel and a supervisor.

There was a comment questioning the willingness of people to work in a radiation situation, especially those from other jurisdictions.

Panel 2 on Capacity to Transport Casualties to Local Treatment Facilities

The presenters on this panel were Richard Alcorta from the Maryland Institute for EMS Systems (National Capital Region); Craig DeAtley from the Washington Hospital Center, Washington, DC (National Capital Region); Bryan Hanley from the Los Angeles County EMS Agency; Douglas Havron from the Southeast Texas Trauma Regional Advisory Council (Houston); and Carl Lindgren from the Arlington Fire Department, Virginia (National Capital Region). They discussed another complication to the limited number of first responders and ambulances relative to the likely number of injured in an IND explosion in a central city as described above. Large cities may have mutual aid arrangements with surrounding communities designed to augment the number of ambulances available in a disaster but many emergency medical technicians (EMTs) and paramedics work for several ambulance services, so there would likely be fewer ambulances than expected because of manning limits.

Also, private-sector EMS personnel do not always have radiation detectors and dosimeters or the level of PPE of their firefighter EMS colleagues in a large city. This would limit their ability to operate in or near the radioactive zone.

Another complication would be "backfill" (i.e., finding personnel to replace the initial responders on a rotating basis as their days of service continue).

Another complication will occur because the sheer number of casualties will necessarily involve EMS from a long distance that have less experience working with a city hit by an IND and perhaps little interoperability. For example, although there may be hundreds of ambulances and thousands of EMTs and paramedics in the National Capital Region, the volume of patients would probably require that many be transported to Baltimore, Richmond, and beyond.

Southern California has developed ambulance strike teams for quick responses to situations requiring the transportation of a large number of people in a short time. An ambulance strike team consists of five ambulances and a leader vehicle carrying communication equipment and supplies. For example, within an hour and a half of the recent San Diego fire, it seemed possible that some hospitals would have to be evacuated, so eight strike teams were mobilized and dispatched on very short notice to be ready in the event this situation would occur.

Big cities generally have a system for balancing the patient load being transported by EMS with the capacity and capability of receiving health care facilities. For example, hospitals in Los Angeles and the surrounding area use a hospital assessment radio system developed by the Healthcare

Association of Southern California. This system, called ReddiNet©, provides real-time data information on bed availability. It has a mass casualty incident screen that, when activated, alerts hospitals with a flashing blue light and an audible alarm that they need to poll their ED beds and their capacity for receiving patients with either life-threatening or minor injuries. Like California, Texas has substate districts for coordinating services. Houston is in a district that uses a catastrophic medical operations center (CMOC) to route EMS-transported patients to an open facility. The CMOC routed 3,300 patients during Hurricanes Katrina and Rita. Northern Virginia has a regional hospital coordination center (RHCC) that assists in determining available resources including hospital beds, operating rooms, staff, medical equipment, supplies, and pharmaceuticals. The RHCC also assists with the allocation of such resources.

One presenter pointed to a likely problem in patient transport. Many people will self-evacuate and go to hospitals to be checked for radiation exposure or be treated for minor injuries, bypassing the field triage system. This may fill hospital EDs even before most ambulances can arrive. On 9/11, for example, the Arlington, Virginia, fire department was told after an hour and a half by one hospital that it was already full and that the ambulances should not bring any more patients, even though the fire department had not transported anyone there for an hour. The hospital was deluged by self-referrals.

A related question is whether roads will be passable if there is a mass "shadow" (unofficial) evacuation by area residents fearful of radiation from fallout. And even if the roads are passable, once the nearby health care facilities fill up, EMS will have to transport patients farther and farther, reducing the turnaround ability of the unit to return for more patients.

Discussion After Panel 2

Most of the discussion following this panel concerned hospital-level issues, such as decontamination procedures, which were addressed by the next panel. Therefore, some of the summary of this part of the discussion appears as part of the discussion following the next panel's presentations.

There was discussion of how to deal with the problem of people transporting themselves to health care facilities with minor injuries or no apparent injuries because they are concerned about possible exposure or contamination. The point was made that this would require "pre-education" of the public or pre-event messaging to inform people about the actual hazards and what steps they could take. It might be suggested, for example, that people take off their outer garments before entering their house and then shower at home rather than appearing at a busy hospital to be decontaminated.

There was also a question about the standards for decontaminating ambulances between runs and after the incident is over.

Panel 3 on Preparedness of the Metropolitan Area's Medical System

Presenters on this panel were Joseph Barbera from the Institute for Crisis, Disaster, and Risk Management at George Washington University; John Brown from the San Francisco EMS Agency; Patricia Hawes from Suburban Hospital, Bethesda, Maryland (National Capital Region); Nathaniel Hupert from Weill Medical College of Cornell University; Amy Kaji from Harbor-UCLA Medical Center, Los Angeles; and Katherine Uraneck from the New York City Department of Health and Mental Hygiene. They described efforts to increase the capacity of hospitals and other health care facilities for the surge of patients that would follow an IND detonation.

Hospital Capacity

Several presenters described how their hospital capacities are shrinking, which in turn reduces their surge capacity in case of a disaster. Los Angeles County, for example, has 74 EMS receiving centers, compared with 91 in 2003. New York City has 65, down 2 from last year. San Francisco has closed one ED and three clinics. The average wait at EDs in Los Angeles County is 6 hours, and "boarding" of patients in the ED is routine because of the chronic hospital bed shortages. As a result, EDs are full. The eight EMS receiving hospitals in San Francisco (one of them a Level 1 trauma center) are on ambulance diversion 1 to 6 days a month. They would be looking to the five adult trauma centers and one pediatric trauma center in the surrounding counties to pick up the overflow.

New York City has approximately 21,000 hospital beds, of which approximately 71 are certified burn beds. In response to a disaster, there is a plan to increase the number of burn beds to 400 by using an additional 30 hospitals, but only for 5 days. The city is working with the state on arrangements to expand access to burn beds statewide. Suburban Hospital in Montgomery County, Maryland, next to Washington, DC, is 1 of 5 hospitals in the county and 34 in the National Capital Region. It is a 250-bed facility with the only trauma center in the county, and it expects to receive up to 40,000 people after a major disaster. After 9/11, Suburban became part of the Bethesda Hospital Emergency Preparedness Partnership with the National Navy Medical Center and NIH Clinical Center in order to share resources and expand capacity.

The Los Angeles County Department of Public Health (LACDPH) used federal HPP funds to establish 13 large hospitals as disaster resource centers (DRCs). DRCs are part of a strategy to enhance surge capacity during disasters through (1) forward deployment of ventilators, pharmaceuticals, medical/surgical supplies, and large tent shelters; and (2) enhanced capacity and cooperation among the 8 to 12 smaller hospitals, clinics, and pre-hospital agencies assigned to each DRC through hospital planning and training. The forward-deployed stockpiles include PPE and 8,000 doses of KI, and in the coming year each DRC will receive 4 or 5 radiation monitoring devices and 100 dosimeters (numbers more suitable for an RDD than an IND event). In 2007, LACDPH acquired a 100-bed mobile hospital, and the state of California has three 200-bed mobile hospitals.

Hupert described a hospital surge model he helped develop with support from the Agency for Healthcare Research and Quality and ASPR. The model has a module for a 1- or 10-kt nuclear device to help health care facilities identify the personnel, equipment, and supplies they would need if there was a detonation. It is available online and includes modules for other types of terrorism, such as an anthrax attack or RDD.[47] Hupert also described a model for a more effective pharmaceutical procurement system for hospitals to use to have more supplies on hand and still average a 3-day supply.

Decontamination

Panelists from several cities discussed plans for the decontamination of patients, although they are training their health care workers that critical care patients must be treated immediately and that, even though 95 percent of any radioactive dust is avoided by simply removing patients' clothes, radiation is going to get into the hospital. Each city has many health care providers, but few have a radiation background or training, and it is difficult to arrange for them to be released for training.

The New York City Department of Health and Mental Hygiene (NYCDOH) has a draft guidance out for comment that provides direction for hospitals responding to a radiological contamination event such as an RDD. The department is developing a plan for mass screening, which would be an enormous undertaking in a city of 8 million. LACDPH has acquired 21 portal radiation monitors that check for radiation as people walk through and thus avoid the need to check each person manually with a radiation detector wand.

Each DRC in Los Angeles County has a trailer with the capacity to decontaminate 50 people an hour for a total of 650 an hour among them. To protect hospital staff, NYCDOH used UASI funds from DHS to purchase area detectors for its EDs, personal digital dosimeters for ED staff,

---

[47] The AHRQ model is at http://hospitalsurgemodel.ahrq.gov/ (accessed June 23, 2009).

and Geiger-Müller survey meters and to provide training in the use of these devices. NYCDOH also provided radiation detectors to EMS units.

The 96 hospitals in the Houston area are equipped and trained to perform Level C decontamination. In the National Capital Region, a committee working through the Metropolitan Council of Governments has conducted an analysis of hospital equipment shortfalls and is standardizing policies and procedures related to decontamination, which it plans to operationalize through training and exercises.

Alternate Care Sites and Altered Standards of Care

The San Francisco Department of Public Health (SFDPH) has designated public libraries and private nonprofit clinics spread across the city to be alternate care sites. There are to be 18 sites, including 6 mobile field care clinics set up next to libraries. The field care clinics are based on the NDMS DMAT model and can treat 50 patients an hour. These mobile clinic alternate care sites would use the mass casualty and austere care protocols used by EMS (described above), and a workgroup is in progress to adapt the austere care protocol to fixed alternate care facilities. SFDPH has also designated casualty collection sites, such as convention centers, in each of its 11 emergency response districts; these sites will be equipped with cots but not medical supplies and equipment.

Countermeasures

Some cities have local stockpiles with pharmaceuticals and medical equipment and supplies. As previously mentioned, LACDPH has distributed stockpiles among its 13 DRCs, but the only radiation countermeasure available at these sites is the 8,000 doses of KI. Similarly, SFDPH has used DHS and HPP funding to establish pharmaceutical caches at each receiving hospital. The caches include antibiotic prophylaxis for a large number of patients in case of a bioterrorist event and for about 1,000 patients for a situation stemming from a radiation, chemical, or conventional explosive event.

Summary

Major cities are working to improve the capacity of their hospitals to respond to the surge of casualties that can be expected in the event of a WMD attack or other disaster, such as an earthquake, hurricane, or pandemic influenza. Their efforts include the establishment of alternate care sites, more detailed triage and treatment protocols for mass casualty events, and regional hospital referral networks. The main driver has been the threats of pandemic influenza and an anthrax or other bioterrorism attack. Recently the cities have been actively preparing for RDD incidents, equipping EMS and EDs with radiation meters and dosimeters and developing policies and procedures for decontamination. However, none claims to be able to accommodate the number of injured that would result from an IND detonation on an emergency basis, let alone to provide definitive care. Hospitals would still have limited supplies on hand and replenishment would be a daunting challenge. The number of intensive care and burn care beds is small in any given metropolitan area relative to the number of trauma, burn, and ARS patients that could be expected; indeed, the number of burn patients from an IND detonation could easily surpass the total number of burn care beds in the United States.

Discussion

There was discussion of plans to have fire departments ready to set up decontamination sites quickly (within 1 to 4 hours) that would generally be able to process 50 people an hour. CDC has suggested the establishment of community reception centers in radiation emergencies, although in an IND event these would likely be in surrounding communities because local health officials would be focusing on treating the immediately injured rather than on decontamination (CDC, 2007). NYCDOH is working on plans for mass screening, which would be an enormous task. For example, for 10,000 people the triage alone would take more than 50 hours of staff time at 20 seconds per person, and decontamination would be even more resource intensive. LACDPH has plans to deploy portal monitors to accommodate larger numbers of people, but contamination of the monitors with radioactive dust and debris could render them useless.

LACDPH is also involving its community health centers. They receive disaster preparedness training, attend DRC meetings, and stockpile supplies.

Victims with burns pose a difficult challenge because they would need care for a long time and not just a quick operation. Given the limited numbers of burn beds in any given area, the focus would be on stabilizing and transferring patients to burn beds throughout the country. As one participant put it, "If the device went off in New York City, would the burn surgeons be ready to provide advice to clinicians in the collar communities around New York City where people are being moved and be ready to accept patients transported to them?" (This is the topic of the next section.)

Panel 4 on Preparedness to Evacuate Serious Casualties from the Metropolitan Area

Presenters on this panel were Joseph Barbera from George Washington University; Dan Hanfling from Inova Health System, Falls Church, Virginia (National Capital Region); Jerome Hauer from the Hauer Group,

Alexandria, Virginia; Aashish Shah from the Texas Department of State Health Services, Houston; and Katherine Uraneck from the New York City Department of Health and Mental Hygiene. Panelists described current and planned arrangements for evacuating the seriously injured victims of an IND detonation to appropriate care settings.

Need for Many Intensive Care Beds for Trauma, Burns, and ARS

Although the number and types of severe acute injuries caused by the immediate effects of a 10-kt IND detonation would depend on a variety of factors, such injuries would most likely number in the thousands to tens of thousands. Many patients would require intensive critical care to survive multiple traumas, severe burns, high doses of prompt irradiation, or some combination of these. No city, even if its health care system was intact and prepared in advance, could treat so many critically ill patients all at once. In an IND attack, however, there would probably be no warning and the health care system—facilities, equipment and supplies, and personnel— would likely be among the casualties as well, leading to reduced capacity.

Hospital capacity limits were just discussed in the previous section. New York City expects to have about 150,000 injured by the initial effects of a 10-kt IND detonation (plus another 300,000 with radiation doses of more than 150 rem [1.5 Sv] from fallout, which would necessitate medical treatment, as discussed in the next section) (Uraneck, 2008). NYCDOH estimates that, under extreme conditions, it could free up between approximately 4,200 and 6,300 beds through early discharge and the canceling of elective procedures, but these would not be critical care beds. As noted above, NYCDOH plans to increase the number of burn beds from 71 to 400 by using an additional 30 hospitals, but they would be available for no more than 5 days. NYCDOH would accomplish this increase by providing burn care training to clinicians and nurses and burn care supply and equipment carts in each of the additional hospitals. Beyond that, the city expects to transfer burn patients to other hospitals outside the area. New York State has developed a health care emergency resource status system that will link with a national system known as HAvBED (National Hospital Available Beds for Emergencies and Disasters) that HHS is developing. On an average day, 35 percent (600) of ICU beds in New York City are unoccupied, but it would be very difficult to increase ICU capacity, especially pediatric, which requires special equipment. Because of a lack of staff, NYCDOH is not counting on additional alternate care sites other than those that will result from expanding treatment areas within existing hospitals. New York City's approach, therefore, will be to evacuate patients once they have received primary or, at least, emergency care. This assumes that means will exist to evacuate a large number of critically ill patients and that there will be places that are prepared to receive them.

Fairfax County, Virginia, immediately west and south of Washington, DC, in the National Capital Region, does not expect to be directly affected by the immediate or longer-term fallout effects of a low-yield IND detonation in Washington, DC. Rather, it expects to be the recipient of large numbers of the injured. Northern Virginia has 12 hospitals, including one Level 1 trauma center, but not a burn center. After 9/11, the anthrax mailings, and the sniper attacks in 2001-2002, the hospitals formed the Northern Virginia Hospital Alliance (NVHA) as a way of developing a regional approach to disaster planning and response.

Another result was the establishment of the Northern Virginia RHCC, a multiagency coordination center responsible for implementing the regional hospital emergency operations plan and the NVHA mutual aid system. The purpose of RHCC is "to ensure patients are delivered to the health care facility most capable of providing definitive patient care, in the shortest and most efficient time possible, through coordination and collaboration with regional partners."

While useful in many mass casualty events, NVHA and RHCC would be quickly overwhelmed by the sheer number of injured needing intensive care after the detonation of an IND, and they would be looking for places to send those patients for the intensity and length of care necessary to survive multiple traumas or ARS. NVHA, like NYCDOH, is concerned about the capacity to move patients and, if they can be moved, whether there will be enough places to treat them.

There is also concern that IND explosions in multiple places, actual or threatened, would make other communities reluctant to send medical help or take patients in case they are the next places hit.

Capacity to Evacuate Patients

Panelist Dan Hanfling asked: Is there a cavalry? The main resource for evacuating the overflow of disaster victims to other hospitals where they can receive necessary care is NDMS, but there was skepticism about whether NDMS has the capacity to move many patients, even though HHS is reviewing the program and increasing its budget. (HHS is asking for $53 million for FY 2009, 14 percent more than the $47 million annual budget it had in FY 2007, when the program was transferred from DHS to HHS.[48])

1. *NDMS medical response teams.* The 55 DMATs and 36 other NDMS medical teams (e.g., burn, pediatric, mental health) would

---

[48] This section draws from studies that Hanfling participated in and cited in his presentation, in particular the study of NDMS by the UPMC Center for Biosecurity (Franco et al., 2007) and the study of national critical care capacity by the Task Force for Mass Casualty Critical Care in 2007 (Christian et al., 2008, and other articles by the task force in the same journal issue).

be sent to disaster sites to augment the capacity of local health care providers in treating patients and stabilizing serious cases for evacuation. Under the best of circumstances (i.e., if the teams can get to the site of an IND event and they are fully manned and equipped when they arrive), the teams would not be operational for a day or two at the earliest (and probably longer) after an IND detonation. Team members would either drive their vehicles or take commercial flights to the nearest open airport.

In sustained operations, a fully operational DMAT can handle about 125 patients a day, including the immediate transfer of 25 patients, stabilization and holding of 6 patients for up to 12 hours, and support of 2 critical-care patients for up to 24 hours.[49] About half of the current 55 DMATs can attain this level of function, with the other DMATs being able to handle a lesser number of patients. If all DMATS were deployed in a mass casualty incident to function as a combined facility for preparing and holding patients for evacuation, they could handle up to 4,200 patients a day (Piggott, 2007).

2. *Patient evacuation.* The second function of NDMS is to move patients to definitive care somewhere in the country. This is carried out by the U.S. Air Force, which can configure large transport aircraft, such as a C-5 Galaxy, C-17 Globemaster, or C-130 Hercules, to transport the patients, who would be accompanied by one of 31 specially trained military medical teams consisting of two flight nurses and three aeromedical technicians. Nineteen of these crews are in the Air Force Reserve and would take time to mobilize. Severely injured patients who are under intravenous treatment, who are taking pain medications or antibiotics, or who are on ventilators would be moved with a three-person Critical Care Air Transport Team, each of which is able to support three patients at once.

In an IND event, the plan would be for DMATs to prepare patients for transport at or near the disaster site. The affected state or states would be responsible for transporting patients from the DMAT staging points to an airport with runways on which military cargo planes could land. At that point the patients would be entered into a military patient-tracking system and flown to a military or other airport near the hospital or hospitals volunteering to taken them. The movement is managed by 1 of about 70 federal coordinating centers (FCCs), which are VA and military medical hospitals responsible for day-to-day coordination of planning and operations in their geographic NDMS patient reception areas.

---

[49] Alternatively, a DMAT can treat 250 ambulatory patients a day or 30-50 patients a day in a standard medical holding-hospital ward setup (Piggott, 2007).

If more aircraft are needed because, for example, the military aircraft are being used for missions overseas, then CRAF, which consists of 1,400 planes available on short notice under contracts with 39 airlines, could be used.

3. *Definitive hospital care.* Some 1,800 hospitals have volunteered more than 100,000 beds in the event of a national disaster. If the beds are used, they will be reimbursed at 110 percent of their Medicare rate. FCCs track patients and transport discharged patients home. However, depending on local circumstances, the hospitals have the option of not providing the volunteered beds.

NDMS was established in 1984, but the first full-scale deployment of its patient evacuation capability did not occur until Hurricane Katrina. At that time several DMAT teams at the New Orleans airport were assigned to triage patients for evacuation by the Air Force. Approximately 4,000 patients were evacuated, about 1,800 by the Air Force and the rest by the National Guard and private planes.

Currently, NDMS is the only available mechanism for providing care to those IND detonation victims who need treatment but who are not able to reach a health care facility in the area that can treat them in a timely way. The explosion of an IND would result in many patients needing critical care in ICUs immediately and many more who would need care during the next few hours and days after being exposed to high doses of radiation from fallout. Currently, NDMS does not have the capacity to handle the number of severely injured patients that can be expected following an IND detonation:

- DMATs and other NDMS medical teams would be able to prepare only a small fraction for evacuation to definitive care sites.
- The capacity to move patients to airports for evacuation by the Air Force would probably be compromised, perhaps severely, in an IND event because of damage to the transportation infrastructure, the crowding of roads still in operation by those self-evacuating, and the possible reluctance of drivers to approach affected areas to pick up passengers. There are only approximately 800 civilian aeromedical helicopters in the country, and they are configured to carry patients in ones or twos.
- At best, Air Force cargo planes could evacuate only a small fraction of the critically injured, even assuming that the planes and medical teams are available, that there is at least one operating airport near the detonation, and that it is possible to transport the patients to the airport by local ambulances, helicopters, or other means, such

as buses. It would take several days for the cargo planes to be configured for stretcher patients and to assemble medical teams.

- It would take 5 days for the first CRAF plane to be converted and arrive.
- Even if 110,000 definitive care beds were available, not enough would be the ICU or burn beds that many IND detonation vic-tims would need. A recent study of ways to expand the number of critical care (i.e., ICU) beds during a surge of patients after a disas-ter showed that increasing the number of beds would be difficult because of a lack of equipment and supplies, especially ventilators, and because of shortages of trained personnel and space. It should be possible, however, to make more effective use of existing national critical care resources to meet a surge by creating better situational awareness of the locations of the beds and by better patient and family tracking (Christian et al., 2008).

Discussion After Panel 4

There was discussion of how health care facilities would be reimbursed for the costs of care to evacuees, some of whom would not have health insurance. Hospitals around the country that take patients through NDMS would be reimbursed 110 percent of their daily rate by the federal Centers for Medicare and Medicaid Services in HHS.

A participant noted that, given the volume of severely injured patients from an IND detonation, there needs to be out-of-the-box thinking about medical transport. Given that the roads would probably be clogged with self-evacuees for several days, other options need to be explored. San Francisco plans to use ferries, for example, and railroads might be used in other areas.

Another participant proposed developing a streamlined process for trans-ferring patients to other health care facilities in an emergency and for keeping track of the patients. If buses are going to be used for additional transport, no standard way exists to configure school buses and passenger buses to be able to accept standard stretchers. Furthermore, there are no procedures for supplying the bus with medications and other supplies, and there are no standard directions to give to the health care workers on the bus.

There was additional discussion about whether health care providers would show up for work or instead would stay away to take care of their families or because they feared exposure to radiation. Again, there is the question whether other states and cities will be willing to dispatch their medi-cal teams to help with an IND event given the risk they might be hit next.

There was discussion of the training and education programs that should be established now for an IND event that may not happen for years.

A participant noted that there is no national locator system that would allow family members and friends to find each other and their children.

Lack of such a system makes some people reluctant to evacuate, and it also poses a burden on health care facilities because people will show up to look for missing family members.

Health care planners are also worried about the consequences of large-scale evacuations by people who are not injured. New York City, for example, expects to have to evacuate 300,000 people for health reasons, but external resources would also have to deal with many times that number of uninjured evacuees who need food, shelter, and regular medical care for their chronic conditions. In addition to a medical crisis involving the injured, there will be an evacuee crisis that could turn into an additional medical crisis. This could be greatly compounded if there were multiple attacks or if people were fleeing other cities in fear of additional attacks.

Shah said that health planners in the Houston area have learned from experience that things do not go according to plan and that the flexibility to respond to unexpected circumstances is the most important capacity to possess. Several years ago Houston went through an exercise of planning for an attack at a sporting event with 100,000 casualties, half seriously ill and half exposed but not ill, and the planners quickly realized that in a real disaster of that magnitude they would not have adequate resources or be able to get them quickly enough. In Houston-Harris County, in response to a series of major hurricanes, a CMOC has been developed, which coordinates bed counts, public health, and, to some degree, private health. Still responses in actual situations are going to be mostly ad hoc despite planning, due to the natural occurrence of unforeseen circumstances.

Hauer listed some things that should work well. DOE's AMS program should have a plane above the plume measuring radiation levels, determining fallout direction, and identifying population exposure. HHS has been working to ensure that DMAT teams will be well equipped and prepared to go wherever they are needed. Someone else mentioned that FEMA has contracted with a company to quickly supply ambulances, helicopters, and paratransit buses with wheelchair lifts in an emergency. The contract calls for moving 3,500 patients within 72 hours. Also, HHS is developing an interactive geographic information system, called MedMap, which will show which medical care sites and assembly center facilities are outside the impact and fallout area and which facilities are available nationally.[50]

---

[50] This was a reference to recent congressional testimony by Rear Admiral W. Craig Vanderwagen, Assistant Secretary of HHS for Preparedness and Response, on HHS's readiness for a radiological or nuclear event. Other federal resources under development cited in Vanderwagen's testimony, but which have not been mentioned before in this report are a federally funded Radiation Laboratory Network; Federal Medical Stations, which are deployable medical facilities able to provide nonacute care and special medical needs sheltering to 250, staffed by rapid deployment force teams from the U.S. Public Health Service commissioned corps; and in collaboration with the American Burn Association, a burn care training course for nurses and a national burn bed tracking system (Vanderwagen, 2008).

Concerning AMS, committee member Fred Mettler pointed out that the Russians had helicopters measuring radiation levels around Chernobyl, but the results did not correspond to ground-level readings close to the failed reactor where the acute fallout was. He suggested that cities deploy perhaps 100 real-time radiation monitoring systems with telemetry and battery backup to locate high-radiation areas after an IND detonation. This would greatly improve the capacity to provide information to the public about whether to shelter in place or to evacuate and could perhaps reduce the amount of self-evacuation and the associated clogging of highways needed to move victims out of the area and medical response teams in.

General Discussion of Topic 7: Preparedness for Responding to the Immediate Casualties of an IND Event

Public Communication

Most of the discussion centered on the need for effective and reliable communication with the public and the mass media, both before an IND event and during the response, and on how to achieve it. The need stems from the scale of the event and the lack of time to prepare. Most people in the immediate aftermath of an IND detonation would have to rely on themselves to make fateful decisions on how best to respond to avoid injury. Also, the more people sheltered in place, the more it would reduce transportation congestion, which would help responders report to work and move patients with serious injuries out to health care facilities. The difficulty is finding a message that will influence people's behavior toward an event that might or might not happen. Some Midwestern cities have worked hard at persuading people to have a personal readiness bag, for example, but they have succeeded in convincing only 25 to 30 percent—perhaps 40 percent at most.

The Homeland Security Institute (HSI) has been working on pre-event and post-event public messaging for a nuclear incident (Box 5). There was some discussion of the difficulty in convincing local media to air public service messages about preparedness for a nuclear event because those in the media believe it will scare people more than help them. HSI is working on a simple message analogous to public safety jingles such as "stop, drop, and roll" and "click it or ticket." One possibility, for example, is "get in, stay in, tune in."

A participant said there seemed to be agreement at the workshop that the pre-event message should be: "Be ready to shelter in place and take care of yourself for an unspecified length of time until it is safe to go outside." This implies that the agencies should have good communications among themselves and agree on a common message before and during an event,

---

BOX 5
Nuclear Incident Communication Planning

The conference report on P.L. 110-28 of 2007 that directed DHS to sponsor the IOM workshop on the current level of medical readiness to respond to a nuclear detonation in Tier 1 UASI cities—summarized in this report—also directed DHS to develop communication plans for responding to a nuclear detonation in Tier 1 UASI cities. DHS assigned that task to HSI. The final report on this task was released in March 2009 (Hampton et al., 2009).

After gathering data from focus groups of members of the public, first-responder workshops, and subject-matter specialists, HSI developed (1) pre-event educational materials for the general public; (2) public messaging templates for use by government leaders at all levels to ensure accuracy and consistency and also build public trust and confidence; and (3) response message templates for use by first responders to address situational awareness, sheltering in place, evacuation, protective actions and medical care, family separations, and the unaffected population. Those materials are presented in appendixes to the final report.

---

but currently there is no guarantee that this will happen. It also implies that there must be a reliable post-event communication system to inform those who are at risk of exposure to radiation and to advise them when the radiation level has fallen to the point that they might consider evacuating. No one claimed to have such a communication system.

Several cities described efforts to inform the media about the effects of a radiological event. Some places have conducted table-top exercises with media representatives responding to anthrax and hurricanes but not IND events. Planners in the National Capital Region are communicating with the *Washington Post*. The Houston Department of Public Health has good relationships with the major news channels and the *Houston Chronicle*, but the emphasis is on the most likely local threats, hurricanes and flooding. A participant suggested that putting the stress on being ready in general, which works for hurricanes and earthquakes, would accomplish much of the purpose of pre-IND event messaging.

Federal Role and State and Local Expectations

There were a number of comments throughout the workshop and during this discussion about encounters with a pervasive fatalistic attitude among many state and local officials that a nuclear explosion would be so overwhelming that local preparations would be able to do little and that they would be waiting for help from the federal government to arrive. One participant said, "I don't think it is that we expect them to come in on a big white horse, but we do hope they don't come slowly trotting in on an old donkey." Local officials should prepare their localities as much as possible for at least the first 3 days and probably for the first week while outside help mobilizes, but eventually only the federal government would have the resources to respond to an event of this scale.

DoD has fewer than 4,000 hospital beds nationwide and would not be able to accommodate many of the injured, but it is very experienced in operational medicine closely tied to supply logistics and personnel management, which is the kind of systematic approach needed in responding to a major disaster. There is some reluctance on DoD's part regarding civil support because the department has a broader mission in national security. After an IND event, in particular, assuming a perpetrator could be identified, DoD forces would likely be mobilized for retaliatory attacks. However, DoD has many facilities and personnel in the continental United States that it must protect. DoD's Guardian facility protection program coordinates with localities where DoD has facilities, either in the locality or adjoining it. The role that military facilities at Walter Reed Army Hospital, Bethesda Naval Hospital, DeWitt Army Hospital at Fort Belvoir, and Andrews Air Force Base play in the National Capital Region provides an example of the cooperation and coordination that can exist between the civilian and military sectors.

It was noted that federal medical and public health preparedness programs—PHEP and HPP—emphasize certain threats but not INDs. It is also difficult to use DHS's state and local grant funding money for medical and public health response. The UASI priority in at least one city is on improving detection, not response.

TOPIC 8: CURRENT PREPAREDNESS TO PREVENT AND TREAT THE DELAYED CASUALTIES OF AN IND EVENT

The participants in this August workshop panel discussion were Thomas Ahrens from the California Department of Public Health, Los Angeles and San Francisco; Brooke Buddemeier from Lawrence Livermore National Laboratory; Kathleen "Cass" Kaufman from the Los Angeles County Department of Public Health; Jeanine Prud'homme from the New York City Department of Health and Mental Hygiene; Irwin Redlener, Columbia University; Adela Salame-Alfie from the New York State Department of Health; Reuben Varghese from Arlington Public Health, Virginia (National Capital Region); and Michael Welling from the Virginia Department of Health (National Capital Region). They addressed the prevention and treatment of the delayed casualties resulting from an IND detonation.

Immediately after an unannounced ground-level burst of a 10-kt IND in the central business district of a major city, some tens of thousands of people would be dead or severely injured. Many more people—some hundreds of thousands—who were not affected by the immediate effects of the explosion would be at risk of injury and death from radioactive fallout but would have the ability to take actions to protect themselves from the radiation. The fallout would begin to fall on the ground, roofs, and vehicles as the winds dispersed it from the mushroom cloud of debris rising up to five miles in the atmosphere. In many cases, these people could reduce or avoid exposure to fallout if they took appropriate steps in the seconds, minutes, or hours after the IND detonation that it would take for the fallout to reach them. The medical response to fallout therefore encompasses both the possibility of prevention of injuries where possible as well as their treatment.

The panel touched on the following issues dealing with local preparedness to prevent and treat "delayed" casualties of an IND detonation:

- Effectiveness of risk communication
- Short- and long-term mental health
- Efficacy of nonmedical protective actions such as sheltering in place and evacuation

Brooke Buddemeier gave the first presentation, a condensed version of his June workshop presentation on fallout effects based on a simulation model of a 10-kt IND detonation in Washington, DC, near the White House. Because many of the participants in the August workshop were not at the June workshop, he reemphasized some of the points he made at that time:

- Fallout would be on the ground quickly, carried by upper atmosphere winds. In this simulation, which used actual weather conditions on May 23, 2005, fallout traveling 75 miles an hour would reach Annapolis in 30 minutes, Delaware in 1 hour, and the Atlantic Ocean in 2 hours. This would make it difficult to escape fallout by evacuating. This would be especially true in the area immediately downwind, where radiation levels could cause severe acute injury in a short period of time.
- Because the biggest particles would drop quickly, the most dangerous fallout would arrive within minutes in an area extending about 9 miles downwind. People would have to seek shelter quickly in order to reduce their exposure and avoid acute injury.
- Buildings offer a significant degree of shielding. For example, the first floor of a typical three-story brick row house in Capitol Hill would cut the 2-hour dose by a factor of 7 from roughly 700 cGy (which few people would survive even with optimum treatment) to

100 cGy (which most people would survive, even without subsequent medical treatment). Being in the basement of such a building would further reduce a person's dose to 10-20 cGy (which would not even cause acute symptoms).

- The radioactivity of fallout decays exponentially with time. For example, a dose rate of 1,500 cGy an hour would fall to 180 cGy an hour within 2 hours and to 7 cGy an hour after 2 days. Sheltering for several hours would greatly decrease a person's dose and in most cases would allow the individual to leave without suffering acute injury.

- About a million people would be in the area in which a 4-day outdoor exposure would lead to 1 cGy or more of dose. This exceeds the DHS and EPA protective action guidance for considering shelter or evacuation (whichever is more effective) to reduce the long-term risk of cancer.

Irwin Redlener was concerned about the general lack of understanding that preparedness for responding to an IND event would save many lives. He contrasted the situation during the Cold War, in which the failure of mutually assured deterrence would have resulted in multiple large nuclear warheads hitting every major city of the United States, with the situation in 2008, when the threat is a "low-yield" IND detonation in one or at most a few cities. Most people in a city hit by an IND would survive, and the number of people who would survive would increase significantly if they knew what steps they should take to protect themselves.

In Redlener's view, the nation is not ready to respond to nuclear terrorism in such a way as to minimize the results of its fallout and other consequences. He identified seven critical barriers to readiness:

1. We have not defined preparedness in order to set goals and measure progress.
2. Preparedness policy, including medical countermeasures, is insufficiently driven by evidence or even by expert consensus. A review of 303 recent articles in the disaster literature found that less than 19 percent were scientific (Abramson et al., 2007).
3. The scale and scope of planning is not adequate for the impact of an IND event.
4. There is insufficient coordination—vertically (between federal, state, and local levels), horizontally (among federal agencies, states, or local health systems), or regionally (among jurisdictions in a metropolitan area). The coordination may be good enough most of the time for responding to hurricanes and tornadoes, but it will not be

good enough for mega-disasters or national security threats. Fallout will cross local and, in some cases, state boundaries, and responding to it will require a regional approach.

5. There is a failure to appreciate the roles, behaviors, and needs of citizens, resulting in a lack of pre-event education about protecting oneself from fallout from an IND detonation, an absence of the capacity for intra- and post-event communication of critical information to people, and a lack of preparedness for a mass evacuation (which will occur naturally but will also be required of those in large areas where fallout is enough to increase future cancer rates).

6. We do not know what "recovery" from nuclear terrorism means, given long-term impacts.

7. The ability of the health care system to respond to an IND event is hampered by underlying problems with insurance coverage, cost of care, an overwhelmed emergency care system, and other systemic problems.

Redlener concluded that improving preparedness for an IND event will require White House leadership, congressional buy-in, and public acceptance.

Reuben Varghese described public health emergency response planning in Arlington, Virginia, a suburb adjoining Washington, DC, and part of the National Capital Region. Arlington is an MMRS city, 1 of 124 in the country that receives grants from DHS of about $200,000 a year to support planning for medical emergencies. Four additional Northern Virginia cities and counties have received UASI funding to conduct MMRS-like activities. For example, the Arlington Public Health Department completed an update of its radiation plan last year. The hope is eventually to have a coordinated region-wide plan for a radiological event. The National Capital Region is also using UASI funding to place GPS units in all Washington, DC, fire and EMS ambulances.

If there were an IND event, Arlington officials expect that the plume would miss the county, in which case the officials would recommend that citizens shelter in place. However, the officials also would expect a mass self-evacuation from Washington, DC. Within 24 to 36 hours, attention would turn to short-term monitoring and decontamination. To do this, the public health department would add a medical component to the public shelters that would be set up by human services under Emergency Support Function #6 (ESF-6) (Mass Care, Housing, and Human Services) and use portal monitors. This would also start the process of long-term monitoring of health effects.

In terms of risk communication and mental health issues, the plan is to have information and to answer questions as soon as possible in order to reduce public anxiety to the greatest degree possible.

Arlington Public Health is uncertain what role the federal government would take during this type of event, which makes planning more difficult. Varghese is concerned about how the region would receive information from the federal level about the size and composition of the IND and on the footprint of the radioactive plume. It would be best if the information were received in a coordinated way, with everyone in the area receiving the same information at the same time.

Michael Welling described how the Division of Radiological Health in the Virginia Department of Health is building on its resources and experience from monitoring nuclear power plants to be the lead state agency in radiation matters. Those at the division expect to be the radiation experts as part of ESF-8 in the Virginia emergency operations center in a disaster, such as an RDD or IND attack.

Welling said the division has been incorporating the National Guard's Weapons of Mass Destruction Civil Support Team (WMD-CST) in its preparedness planning and nuclear power plant exercises. He recommended that other states do the same with their WMD-CSTs.

In 2008 the division acquired a mobile laboratory equipped to survey radiation. The vehicle also contains an incident command communications system. The division employs Hotspot, a computer program developed by Lawrence Livermore National Laboratory that can produce atmospheric dispersion (i.e., plume) models, which are designed primarily for field use by emergency responders to incidents involving the release of radioactive materials, such as would occur in a nuclear power plant accident.

Thomas Ahrens described the roles and capabilities of the California Department of Public Health in an IND event. The strategy at the state level is to take on the medical logistics of finding, locating, and procuring medical supplies and pharmaceuticals and getting them to the people in need in the affected area. Afterward, as people are transported out of the area and possibly around the country for further diagnosis and treatment, the plan calls for tracking them and making sure that adequate supplies are provided to them. The main way that the state addresses the medical logistics issue is to coordinate closely with the SNS program. Ahrens said California has a fairly robust system that includes state and private caches of pharmaceuticals and medical supplies as well as the SNS program. Also, California has instituted a step-wise process in which requests for medical assistance and materiel originate locally and are combined at the regional level (California is divided into six regions for emergency response purposes), and then go to the state level where they are combined again to ensure that there are no duplicate or unnecessary requests before a request goes to the SNS program.

California also maintains relationships with the National Guard, CDC, DOE, and others who will serve as responders and sources of expert advice in the event of an IND detonation or other emergency. These involve participation in drills as well as other forms of collaborative planning. Ahrens suggested the use of no-notice drills to test the system. For example, a no-notice tabletop drill involving calls to the Guard or DOE could be used to discern what assets these agencies would provide in such a situation.

California is also working with Rx Response, a cooperative program among pharmaceutical manufacturers and suppliers, pharmacy groups, and others that will provide a single source of information in the event of a disaster. The Rx Response program was placed on alert during the recent California forest fires, for example.

California is generally taking an all-hazards approach to preparedness, although plans have been developed for anthrax, pandemic influenza, smallpox, and other specific threats. The state has a set of standing emergency resource contracts to supply various items such as trucks to move medical equipment and supplies.

One problem facing the state is the short shelf life of pharmaceuticals in its stockpile. ARS treatments, such as cytokines and other blood products, have a shelf life of 30 months and are costly. The SNS program has the authority to extend expiration dates of pharmaceuticals in its stockpile, but the states do not, which makes it very expensive to maintain a non-federal stockpile. Also, California is concerned about the adequacy of the supply of cytokines, which now are only made for treatment of cancer and hematological disorders.

Jeanine Prud'homme provided a summary of preparedness plans and programs related to nuclear and radiological threats in New York City. After 9/11, recognizing the need to dedicate full-time staff and activities to CBRNE preparedness, NYCDOH established the Bureau of Environmental Emergency Preparedness and Response. New York City has a CIMS modeled after the national Incident Command System. In a CBRNE incident believed or suspected of being a terrorist event, the police department would be the designated incident commander. The fire department would be responsible for life safety and public decontamination operations under CIMS. In a radiological or IND event, under the city's Radiation Emergency Operations Plan, NYCDOH would be responsible for medical and mental health activities, environmental mitigation, health risk assessment, and public health communications. Responding to a radiological or nuclear event would demand a coordinated regional response. Recognizing this, the partners in the New York Securing the Cities program—the New York City police, fire, health, and environmental protection departments; the Port Authority of New York/New Jersey; the Metropolitan Transportation Authority; the states of New York, New Jersey, and Connecticut; and four surrounding New York counties—intend to form a regional radiological response and recovery subcommittee.

Securing the Cities is a DHS grant program for high-threat metropolitan areas to support regional capabilities in the detection and interdiction of illicit radioactive materials. The New York City metropolitan area, including its ports, was selected to be the pilot program. Except for the radiological response and recovery subcommittee, Securing the Cities is focused solely on heading off an attack, not on the consequences of a successful attack.

As in other cities, the initial preparedness effort is focused on radiological, not nuclear, threats. Once the plans for a radiological attack are in place, New York will address nuclear preparedness.

Prud'homme listed some gaps, in addition to the lack of fully coordinated regional response capability in the New York metropolitan area that need to be addressed by local and regional efforts:

- Lack of guidance for choosing a sheltering-in-place versus evacuation response to an IND or other radiological event
- Lack of open-source information on what conditions will be like after an IND detonation, which is needed for realistic response planning
- The need for better systems for real-time data collection and interpretation
- The need for a robust tiered communications system
- The need for mitigation and recovery plans for radiological contamination in an urban environment

---

Cass Kaufman said that Los Angeles County, like New York City, is planning to use the multiagency radiation response plan it has developed as the basis of a nuclear response plan, while recognizing that a nuclear detonation will have some unique aspects. In a radiological incident, the PAG limits are an accumulated dose of 50 rem (500 mSv) for lifesaving and an accumulated dose of 10 rem (100 mSv) for protecting critical emergency response-related infrastructure. Los Angeles County is looking at the need to increase these limits significantly for responders in a nuclear detonation event.

For enhanced situational awareness, all staff members carry radiation meters with a GPS in their vehicles. The readings are automatically sent wirelessly to populate a real-time electronic map of radiation levels around Los Angeles County. If there was a radiation incident alert, staff members would form into teams and drive toward the incident until they hit 100 millirem per hour on their instruments. This would help define the radioactive zone on the map. The same response would be taken for an IND event, except that the staff members might have to drive *out* to find the 100 millirem per hour perimeter, depending on where they were when the device went off. The Los Angeles County Sheriff and Los Angeles Police Department helicopters also have radiation detectors, and there are plans to link these data into the map. By the time federal assets, such as the Phase 1 FRMAC team, arrived, Los Angeles County would have real-time data on the footprint of the plume that could be plugged into the FRMAC dispersion model.

Los Angeles County also has its own stockpile of chelating agents and KI it can use for responders before the SNS arrives.

All Los Angeles County radiation exercises include mental health. Mental health personnel have received training on radiation, and LACDPH staff have been briefed on the kinds of psychological effects that they can expect to experience as a way of preparing them for a radiological event.

LACDPH has pre-scripted public information announcements for an RDD incident. A first draft was written by a radiation expert for technical accuracy. Then the county psychiatrist revised the draft so that the message would be better understood by the public. For example, the phrase "first responders" was changed to "police and fire rescue" for clarity, and the open-ended statement "we will get back to you when we have more information" was changed to give a specific time in order to reduce public anxiety. The announcements would have to be modified for an IND event.

Adele Salame-Alfie reviewed the roles of the New York State Department of Health (NYSDOH) in any IND event. The department has the lead role at the state level in responding to radiological emergencies involving such incidents as nuclear power plant accidents, accidents during the transport of radiological materials, and now terrorist attacks with RDDs or INDs. The department is represented on the New York Securing the Cities radiological response and recovery subcommittee, but its main emphasis is on training local health departments and emergency management in the counties that have little radiological response capacity (i.e., those outside the New York metropolitan area and without nuclear power plants). In the event an RDD or IND was detonated, NYSDOH would be involved in a range of activities, including field sampling and analysis, dose assessment, and implementation of protective action guidelines. It would provide assistance with population monitoring and public information. The SNS would come to the state initially and be distributed by NYSDOH, and the department would advise on the use of medical countermeasures.

In May and June 2009 the New York State Capital District area—Albany and Rensselaer counties—will host a full-scale FRMAC response exercise involving an RDD. It will begin with a 2-day tabletop exercise to simulate the first 48 hours (mostly local and state activities since the scenario assumes that federal assistance will not arrive for 2 or 3 days) and will be followed by a 3-day full-scale exercise including federal agencies.

Discussion of Preparedness to Prevent and Treat the Delayed Casualties of an IND Detonation

The discussion addressed a number of areas in which preparedness policies and procedures are not clear.

Sheltering in Place or Evacuation

This question was posed: Who will decide to recommend sheltering or evacuation and on what basis? Currently, each area is deciding what to do. In Los Angeles County, for example, the initial message to those within a half-mile or mile of the detonation point will be to shelter in place because levels of radioactivity outdoors will be too high for them or rescuers to be outdoors for a day or two. Meanwhile, Los Angeles will be conducting flyovers to map the areas and levels of radiation, to determine when and where it is safe to evacuate people. Outside the close-in area, Los Angeles County will use the EPA PAGs, which call for evacuation if the 4-day dose is expected to be 1 rem (10 mSv) or more. Since this would involve a large number of people and result in significant traffic congestion, the county will attempt to have people shelter in place for several days until it can arrange for buses. New York City would also use the PAGs, but it sees the problem to be lack of information on which to estimate the dose levels.

This discussion of sheltering and evacuation policies was intertwined with the public messaging topic, which is summarized below.

Pre-Event and Intra-Event Messaging

A participant posed the issue as follows: "If you don't get public messaging correct in the first 12 or 24 hours in a post-detonation environment, you are going to wind up with another 100,000 or 200,000 people stuck on the roads who are now going to become fallout victims." The actual numbers would depend on circumstances, but whatever the number, automobiles would provide little shielding to the passengers inside from fallout on the ground around them.

Others pointed out that messaging during an event would probably have little impact without some pre-event education that was understandable to people. For example, NYSDOH found in preparing training courses for local health departments that the phrase "shelter in place" was not understood by most people.

Another factor identified was the need for the information to come from a credible source. CDC has found in its research on crisis and risk communication that the more local the source, the more credible it is for the public. This implies the need for the identification and preparation of local subject matter specialists who can put out the messages.

Several participants had been involved in workshops on messaging for an IND event held by HSI in four cities during 2008, which examined messages such as "go in, stay in, tune in," but the results had not yet been published.[51] The Conference of Radiation Control Program Directors (CRCPD) is also working on messaging, beginning with a comprehensive review of messages that have been developed by various groups and localities.[52]

CDC also found that the public and clinicians need different messages. A participant suggested having emergency preparedness be part of continuing education requirements for clinicians. At least one state requires a certain number of hours of emergency preparedness education.

Decontamination Criteria and Policies

Another area of extended discussion was how to deal with radiation contamination of people, especially uninjured people needing food and shelter and medical care for chronic conditions. The Red Cross, the lead for ESF-6, the "Mass Care, Housing, and Human Services" annex to the NRF, has a zero-contamination policy for entry into shelters. This poses a major problem because many people will be sufficiently contaminated to trigger portal monitor alarms, and it will not be possible to decontaminate hundreds of thousand of people in 12 hours. Many contaminated individuals will have chronic medical conditions that may be exacerbated if they do not receive shelter, food, and medical care. There were suggestions that removal of clothing and washing of face and hands would be adequate even if it did not provide 100 percent decontamination and that there could be agreement on a low but nonzero level of contamination at which to set the portal monitor alarms.

Health care providers who treated victims of the Chernobyl reactor

---

[51] The HSI report was published in March 2009 (Hampton et al., 2009). See Box 5 for a brief summary.

[52] In December 2008, CRCPD published a report on keys to successful radiological response (CRCPD, 2008).

accident received at most 1 rad (1 cGy). Even the rescuers at Chernobyl breathing the dust received less than 10 percent of their dose from internal contamination.

Pre- and intra-event messaging would be important in allaying public fears that contamination would be a major hazard and lessening the fears of health care providers that treating trauma patients would put them at risk of being contaminated.

Identifying the Acutely Irradiated

An IND explosion could irradiate upwards of 100,000 people to several hundred rad (cGy) or more. Two hundred rad (cGy) is the fatality threshold at which about 5 percent of those exposed would die without treatment. Currently, as discussed earlier in this report, dose assessment for initial field triage purposes is assessed by performing an evaluation that includes determining where the person was at the time of detonation and estimating the time from irradiation until he or she vomited as well as other, less reliable symptoms such as erythema. At the hospitals, laboratory tests (e.g., serial complete blood counts) would be useful but the capacity to conduct laboratory tests would be severely limited relative to demand.

The problem of identifying and transporting people with radiation injuries would be complicated because many of them would be in areas of heavy fallout and infrastructure destruction where for several days after the explosion it would be dangerous and difficult for EMS to operate.

Addressing Long-Term Effects

This topic was not a focus of the workshop, but it was touched on a number of times, in part because it involves activities that should begin immediately after an IND is detonated. A large number of people, upwards of one million, would likely have been in areas where the 4-day fallout dose was 1 rem (10 mSv) or more. Although doses of 1 to 5 rem (10 to 40 mSv) are estimated to increase the long-term cancer rate slightly, the absolute number of people potentially affected by such a low dose could be several thousand.[53]

Because these people would not be acutely affected, the plans would be to receive and maintain them in shelters until it is safe for them to return to their homes. Los Angeles County's playbook, for example, calls for registration at ESF-6 shelters. This would probably be piggybacked on their point

---

[53] According to González (2005), each mSv would increase the probability of cancer in the long term by 0.005 percent. Assuming the average dose in the area exposed to between 10 and 50 mSv is 30 mSv, the probability would be 0.15 percent (0.0005 times 30), which would affect approximately 1,500 of a population of one million.

of dispensing database by adding information to the database, especially details about where the person was at the time of detonation and time to vomiting, in order to estimate the person's dose.

Administering Countermeasures

The question posed was about the criteria for administering decorporating and blocking agents such as DTPA. With respect to the decorporating and blocking agents, a major problem is determining how much internal contamination someone has experienced.

Another question was about the adequacy of the supply of cytokines such as filgrastim. Hospitals would only have a small supply on hand for treating oncology and hematology patients. The Public Health Emergency Medical Countermeasures Enterprise has a requirement for 200,000 treatment courses of a medical countermeasure to mitigate or treat the neutropenia associated with ARS. Currently, SNS includes a modest quantity of filgrastim in its vendor-managed inventory system. HHS is currently seeking to increase its stockpile of medical countermeasures for hematopoietic syndrome and radiation-induced neutropenia.

WRAP-UP AND FINAL THOUGHTS

Committee chair Georges Benjamin concluded the workshop by summarizing the main points he had heard during the presentations and discussions. First, the detonation of an IND would be a national catastrophe of unprecedented proportions because of the large number of casualties, reinforced by the social, economic, and psychological impacts. Local and state responses would be overwhelmed immediately, and it would be several days or a week before federal and other resources could be fully mobilized. HHS has developed a playbook outlining how the federal medical response to an IND detonation would evolve and unfold and intends to publish this on the Internet.

Second, it was apparent from the presentations that there are many emergency preparedness efforts going on at multiple levels, and the degree of planning varies among them. Generally, large urban areas and their states have begun to prepare their responses to a radiological event such as an RDD but are only beginning to think about what they should do to prepare for a possible IND detonation. The workshop brought up some important decisions that must be resolved, such as radiation exposure limits for emergency responders and the public and also the criteria for telling the populace to shelter where they are or to evacuate (discussed below).

Third, many federal agencies are poised to help, but there is a lack of awareness at the local level about what assets would be available and the process.[54] More planning and exercising for an IND detonation contingency is needed at the local level if local and state planners are to understand how these various pieces would fit together in an actual event.

Fourth, in addition to the lack of knowledge of federal plans and resources for responding to an IND event, localities and states generally lack awareness of the number and mix of casualties that would occur in plausible detonation scenarios. There is currently little open-source information on the conceivable conditions following an IND detonation in a modern U.S. city. The information provided by Brooke Buddemeier in his presentation at the June workshop is all that is public, and it did not include estimates of the numbers of casualties by type of injury except in the most general terms (i.e., "hundreds of thousands of casualties can occur from the prompt effects in the first few minutes within a few miles of detonation site" and "hundreds of thousands of acute casualties from radioactive fallout can occur within 15 km downwind"). This makes it difficult for localities and states to plan their responses.[55]

Fifth, there are significant limitations on the effectiveness of a response. Current supplies of specific (e.g., cytokines) and nonspecific (e.g., blood products) medical countermeasures are not matched to the projected requirements of an IND detonation, and the logistical challenges that would have to be overcome in order to administer these countermeasures when they are needed are substantial. There will not be enough vehicles and airplanes to extricate victims and move them to treatment facilities.

Sixth, the nation is not prepared to respond to the medical and public health consequences of an IND detonation, but it is not clear what "prepared" means. Preparedness is a process, not a point in time, and it is not clear what the goal should be. Determining such a goal would help in measuring and evaluating progress toward preparedness.

---

[54] As footnoted earlier, HHS's nuclear detonation playbook, which would lay out the various roles and responsibilities of the federal agencies in more detail, has not yet (as of June 23, 2009) been released.

[55] Some additional information has been released since the workshops were held, cited in footnotes 13 and 16 and Box 1. Buddemeier (2008) has estimated the unduplicated number of injured from all prompt effects (blast, thermal, and radiation) in his Washington, DC, scenario as 250,000, divided into those who (1) would recover without advanced medical aid, (2) would succumb to fatal doses of radiation or combinations of injuries in the coming weeks and months, and (3) would most benefit from advanced medical aid. He added that the number injured by prompt effects in New York City would be larger, about 400,000. In January 2009, the Homeland Security Council issued *Planning Guidance for Response to a Nuclear Detonation*, which provides information about the detonation effects of a 10-kt IND in an urban environment and advice on effective response strategies for state and local responders to use (EOP, 2009). Law et al. (2008) analyzed alternative sheltering and evacuation strategies in the fallout area, finding that sheltering for a period of time immediately after a detonation, followed by delayed evacuation when radiation levels have declined, is generally the best strategy.

Seventh, many important strategic decisions have to be made at the national (i.e., combined local, state, and federal) level:

- How to inform and engage the public in the process of deciding what responses would be realistic and appropriate.
- What the triage criteria and process should be, given the mismatch between medical needs and resources: HHS is developing a system, but it is not clear what it will be or how it will be legitimated among providers and the public.
- What the radiation exposure levels for responders should be, and who should apply them: Should each state or locality decide for its people, or should there be national consensus standards?
- Whether to tell the public to shelter in place or evacuate, and on what criteria to base such a decision: For reasons discussed during the workshop (e.g., the speed of the arrival of fallout and the relatively effective protection that can be provided by buildings versus the probability of gridlock), the default policy probably should be, "Shelter in place until we let you know it is safe enough to evacuate," but no one has stated this officially. Part of the problem is that this or any other blanket policy will not be the best policy for every situation, but the capacity to provide more nuanced advice probably does not exist at this time. No blanket policy is perfect, but the capacity to provide tailored advice during an event is and will continue to be quite limited.
- To what extent plume models should form the basis of decisions to recommend that people should shelter or evacuate: There was evidence presented at the workshop that the footprint of the fallout might well be patchy rather than the sharply defined cigar or fan shape provided by plume models, because the winds at different levels might be going in different directions and shifting at the same time.
- How long-term medical effects should be handled: This was not addressed at the workshop, but steps must be taken soon after the event to identify people exposed to 1 rem (10 mSv) or more, inform them of the long-term risks of cancer, and implement registries to keep track of them. There will also be long-term mental health and behavioral effects that will need to be monitored. DoD has been developing instruments and procedures for military personnel serving in Iraq and Afghanistan that might be transferable into the civilian setting.
- How to manage public and health care professional concerns and fear: There is no clear strategy for communicating with people and keeping them informed, especially vulnerable populations who have fewer resources to help them make it through a devastating event.

Eighth, there are few medical countermeasures available for victims of radiation exposure, and more are greatly needed. Current licensed countermeasures are limited to decorporation and blocking agents, but internal contamination with radionuclides will not be a significant determinant of near-term morbidity and mortality in an IND scenario.

Radioiodine is not likely to be a major fission product of an IND, and in any case, KI works best when taken before exposure and has little effect unless it is applied within a day or two after exposure, which will be difficult to accomplish. In any event, ingestion is not likely to be a major problem in the days after an IND detonation, although eventually it will become one as people began to ingest contaminated food and water.

The standard treatment for ARS includes cytokines, antibiotics, and other supportive care. New countermeasures are under development as part of a concerted federal effort, with some products in comparatively late stages of development or licensed for other indications. However, none have yet been licensed for the treatment of radiation injury and current federal investment for the development of such products is limited in comparison with that for biodefense countermeasures.

Also, radiation countermeasures are not going to help people injured by the blast and burn effects if they do not receive trauma care, which poses a great challenge for the reasons mentioned throughout the workshop and described above (e.g., lack of health care facilities, especially for burn patients and other patients needing specialized intensive care; limited assets for moving patients to existing health care facilities, regionally and nationally; problems with the resupply of health care facilities that have one-day inventories of drugs and other supplies).

Finally, while no preparations could fully mitigate the impacts of a nuclear detonation in the middle of a major U.S. city, the workshop discussions touched on a number of ways that governments at all levels have begun to improve their capacity to respond to such an event, especially by increasing joint information sharing and response planning on a regional basis. Determining how much priority to give such efforts, considering the more likely threats of the occurrence of events such as earthquakes, hurricanes, and other forms of terrorism, was beyond the committee's charge. However, many of these efforts would also help improve the nation's capacity to respond to other types of mass casualty events.

REFERENCES

Abramson, D. M., S. S. Morse, A. L. Garrett, and I. Redlener. 2007. Public health disaster research: Surveying the field, defining its future. *Disaster Medicine and Public Health Preparedness* 1(1):57-62.

AFRRI (Armed Forces Radiobiology Research Institute). 2003. *Medical management of radiological casualties, 2nd edition.* Bethesda, MD: Author. http://www.afrri.usuhs.mil/ www/outreach/pdf/2edmmrchandbook.pdf (accessed June 23, 2009).

Alt, L. A., C. D. Forcino, and R. I. Walker. 1989. Nuclear events and their consequences. In *Textbook of military medicine, Part I, Vol. 2, Medical consequences of nuclear warfare,* edited by R. I. Walker and T. J. Cerveny. Washington, DC: Office of the Surgeon General, Department of the Army. http://www.bordeninstitute.army.mil/published_volumes/ nuclearwarfare/chapter1/chapter1.pdf (accessed June 23, 2009).

Bader, J. L., J. Nemhauser, F. Chang, B. Mashayekhi, M. Sczcur, A. Knebel, C. Hrdina, and N. Coleman. 2008. Radiation Event Medical Management (REMM): Website guidance for health care providers. *Prehospital Emergency Care* 12(1):1-11.

Becker, S. M. 2004. Emergency communication and information issues in terrorism events involving radioactive materials. *Biosecurity and Bioterrorism* 2:195-207.

Becker, S. M. 2007. Communicating risk to the public after radiological incidents. *British Medical Journal* 335(7630):1106-1107.

Becker, S. M. 2009. Preparing for terrorism involving radioactive materials: Three lessons from recent experience and research. *Journal of Applied Security Research* 4(1):9-20.

Becker, S. M., and S. A. Middleton. 2008. Improving hospital preparedness for radiological terrorism: Perspectives from emergency department physicians and nurses. *Disaster Medicine and Public Health Preparedness* 2(3):174-184.

Bell, W. C., and C. E. Dallas. 2007. Vulnerability of populations and the urban health care systems to nuclear weapon attack—examples from four American cities. *International Journal of Health Geographics* 6:5. http://www.ij-healthgeographics.com/content/ pdf/1476-072X-6-5.pdf (accessed June 23, 2009).

Buddemeier, B. 2008. *Improving response to the aftermath of radiological and nuclear terrorism.* Publication number LLNL-PRES-404937-rev1. Presentation at the 2008 Bio-Dose Conference, Hanover, NH, September 8.

Buddemeier, B., and M. Dillon. Forthcoming. *Key response planning factors for response to the aftermath of nuclear terrorism.* Publication number LLNL-TR-410067. Livermore, CA: Lawrence Livermore National Laboratory.

Bunn, M., A. Wier, and J. Holdren. 2003. *Controlling nuclear warheads and materials: A report card and action plan.* Project on Managing the Atom, Harvard University. http:// www.nti.org/e_research/cnwm/cnwm.pdf (accessed June 23, 2009).

CDC (Centers for Disease Control and Prevention). 2007. *Population monitoring in radiation emergencies: A guide for state and local public health planners.* http://emergency.cdc. gov/radiation/pdf/population-monitoring-guide.pdf (accessed June 23, 2009).

Chaffee, M. 2009. Willingness of health care personnel to work in a disaster: An integrative review of the literature. *Disaster Medicine and Public Health Preparedness* 3(1):42-56.

Christian, M. D., A. V. Devereaux, J. R. Dichter, J. A. Geiling, and L. Rubinson. 2008. Definitive care for the critically ill during a disaster: Current capabilities and limitations: From a Task Force for Mass Critical Care summit meeting, January 26-27, 2007, Chicago. *Chest* 133(5):8S-17S.

Coleman, C. N., C. Hrdina, J. L. Bader, A. Norwood, R. Hayhurst, J. Forsha, K. Yeskey, and A. Knebel. 2008. Medical response to a radiologic/nuclear event: Integrated plan from the Office of the Assistant Secretary for Preparedness and Response, Department of Health and Human Services. *Annals of Emergency Medicine* 53(2):213-222. http://download. journals.elsevierhealth.com/pdfs/journals/0196-0644/PIIS0196064407018999.pdf (accessed June 23, 2009).

Collins, D. L. 2002. Human responses to the threat of or exposure to ionizing radiation at Three Mile Island, Pennsylvania, and Goiânia, Brazil. *Military Medicine* 167(2 Suppl): 137-138.

Commission on the Prevention of Weapons of Mass Destruction Proliferation and Terrorism. 2008. *World at risk: The report of the Commission on the Prevention of WMD Proliferation and Terrorism.* New York: Vintage Books. http://www.preventwmd.gov/report/ (accessed June 23, 2009).

Cone, D. C., and B. A. Cummings. 2006. Hospital disaster staffing: If you call, will they come? *American Journal of Disaster Medicine* 1(1):28-36.

CRCPD (Conference of Radiation Control Program Directors). 2008. *Report on the CDC-CRCPD roundtable on communication and teamwork: Keys to successful radiological response.* Frankfort, KY: Author. http://www.crcpd.org/CDC/ReportOnCDC-CRCPD_ RoundtableOnCommunicationAndTeamwork.pdf (accessed June 23, 2009).

Dallas, C. 2008. *Impact of small nuclear weapons on Washington, DC: Outcomes and emergency response recommendations.* Prepared statement prepared for "Nuclear Terrorism: Confronting the Challenges of the Day After," hearing held by the Senate Committee on Homeland Security and Governmental Affairs, April 15. http://hsgac.senate.gov/ public/_files/041508Dallas.pdf (accessed June 23, 2009).

Dallas, C. E., and W. C. Bell. 2007. Prediction modeling to determine the adequacy of medical response to urban nuclear attack. *Disaster Medicine and Public Health Preparedness* 1(2):80-89.

DHS (Department of Homeland Security). 2006. Protective action guides for radiological dispersal device (RDD) and improvised nuclear device (IND) incidents. *Federal Register* 71(1):174-196. http://edocket.access.gpo.gov/2006/pdf/05-24521.pdf (accessed June 23, 2009).

DHS. 2008. Planning guidance for protection and recovery following radiological dispersal device (RDD) and improvised nuclear device (IND) incidents. *Federal Register* 73(149): 45029-45048. http://www.fema.gov/good_guidance/download/10260 (accessed June 23, 2009).

EOP (Executive Office of the President). 2009. *Planning guidance for response to a nuclear detonation.* First edition, January 16. Developed by the Interagency Policy Coordination Subcommittee for Preparedness & Response to Radiological and Nuclear Threats. http:// www.epa.gov/radiation/docs/er/planning-guidance-response-nuclear-detonation-FINAL. pdf (accessed June 23, 2009).

EPA (Environmental Protection Agency). 1992. *Manual of protective action guides and protective actions for nuclear incidents.* EPA 400-R-92-001. http://www.epa.gov/rpdweb00/ docs/er/400-r-92-001.pdf (accessed June 23, 2009).

Florig, H. K., and B. Fischhoff. 2007. Individuals' decisions affecting radiation exposure after a nuclear explosion. *Health Physics* 92(5):475-483.

Franco, C., E. Toner, R. Waldhorn, T. V. Inglesby, and T. O'Toole. 2007. The National Disaster Medical System: Past, present, and suggestions for the future. *Biosecurity and Bioterrorism* 5(4):319-325. http://www.upmc-biosecurity.org/website/resources/publications/ 2007_orig-articles/2007-12-04-natldisastermedsystempastpresfut.html (accessed June 23, 2009).

Glasstone, S., ed. 1962. *The effects of nuclear weapons, revised edition.* Washington, DC: U.S. Government Printing Office. [This edition has a chapter on "Principles of Protection" that was not in the 1977 edition.]

Glasstone, S., and P. J. Dolan, eds. 1977. *The effects of nuclear weapons, third edition.* Washington, DC: U.S. Government Printing Office. http://www.princeton.edu/sgs/publications/articles/ effects/ (accessed June 23, 2009).

González, A. J. 2005. Radiation protection in the aftermath of a terrorist attack involving exposure to ionizing radiation. *Health Physics* 89(5):418-446.

Hampton, B., B. Altmire, B. Brunjes, D. M. Jennings, W. B. Mallory, S. Maloney, and R. Tuohy. 2009. *Nuclear incident communication planning—final report.* Prepared for the Department of Homeland Security, Office of Health Affairs. Arlington, VA: Homeland Security Institute.

Helfand, I., L. Forrow, and J. Tiwari. 2002. Nuclear terrorism. *British Medical Journal* 324(7333):356-359. http://www.bmj.com/cgi/reprint/324/7333/356.pdf (accessed June 23, 2009).

IOM (Institute of Medicine). 1999. *Potential radiation exposure in military operations: Protecting the soldier before, during, and after.* Committee on Battlefield Radiation Exposure Criteria, F. A. Mettler, Jr., Chairman, and S. Thaul and H. O'Maonaigh, eds. Washington, DC: National Academy Press.

Kessler, R. C., G. Andrews, L. J. Colpe, E. Hiripi, D. K. Mroczek, S. L. Normand, E. E. Walters, and A. M. Zaslavsky. 2002. Short screening scales to monitor population prevalences and trends in non-specific psychological distress. *Psychological Medicine* 32(6):959-976.

Kreisher, O. 2008. Military forms special units to respond to possible WMD attacks. *Government Executive.* December 17. http://www.govexec.com/story_page.cfm?articleid=41650 (accessed June 23, 2009).

Lanzilotti, S. S., D. Galanis, N. Leoni, and B. Craig. 2002. Hawaii medical professionals assessment. *Hawaii Medical Journal* 61(8):162-173.

Law, K., T. West, L. Brandt, and A. Yoshimura. 2008. *Shelter-evacuate strategies and consequences following an urban nuclear detonation.* Presentation at 53rd Annual Meeting of the Health Physics Society, Pittsburgh, PA, July 13-17. http://birenheide.com/hps/2008program/singlesession.php3?sessid=WAM-B (accessed June 23, 2009).

Levi, M. 2007. *On nuclear terrorism.* Cambridge, MA: Harvard University Press.

Marrs, R. E. 2007. *Radioactive fallout from terrorist nuclear detonations.* Lawrence Livermore National Laboratory Report No. UCRL-TR-230908. https://e-reports-ext.llnl.gov/pdf/347266.pdf (accessed June 23, 2009).

Morgan, M. G., B. Fischhoff, A. Bostrom, and C. J. Atman. 2002. *Risk communication: A mental models approach.* New York: Cambridge University Press.

NCRP (National Council on Radiation Protection and Measurements). 2005. *Key elements of preparing emergency responders for nuclear and radiological terrorism.* NCRP Commentary No. 19. Bethesda, MD: NCRP.

Nightingale, S. L., J. M. Prasher, and S. Simonson. 2007. Emergency Use Authorization (EUA) to enable use of needed products in civilian and military emergencies, United States. *Emerging Infectious Diseases* 13(7):1046-1051. http://www.cdc.gov/eid/content/13/7/pdfs/1046.pdf (accessed June 23, 2009).

Norris, F. H., J. L. Hamblen, L. M. Brown, and J. A. Schinka. 2008. Validation of the Short Posttraumatic Stress Disorder Rating Interview (expanded version, Sprint-E) as a measure of postdisaster distress and treatment need. *American Journal of Disaster Medicine* 3(4):201-212.

Piggott, W. J. 2007. *National Disaster Medical System (NDMS).* PowerPoint presentation by the NDMS Western Medical Director to the Bureau of Public Health Emergency Preparedness & Response, Arizona Department of Health Services. http://www.azdhs.gov/phs/edc/edrp/es/pdf/ndms_piggott.pdf (accessed June 23, 2009).

Prasanna, P. G. S., R. E. Berdychevski, K. Krasnopolsky, G. K. Livingston, M., Moroni, P. R. Martin, H. Romm, U. Subramanian, R. C. Wilkins, and M. A. Yoshida. 2008. *Radiation cytogenetic biosimetry laboratory automation and inter-laboratory comparison of the dicentric assay.* Abstract of presentation at BioDose 2008, Hanover, NH, September 9, 2008. http://www.dartmouth.edu/~eprctr/biodose2008/pdf/PellmarWilkins1.pdf (accessed June 23, 2009).

Quereshi, K., R. R. Gershon, F. M. Sherman, T. Straub, E. Gebbie, M. McCollum, M. J. Erwin, and S. S. Morse. 2005. Health care workers' ability and willingness to report to duty during catastrophic disasters. *Journal of Urban Health* 82(3):378-388.

RERF (Radiation Effects Research Foundation). 2002. *Reassessment of the atomic bomb radiation dosimetry for Hiroshima and Nagasaki—dosimetry system 2002.* Hiroshima, Japan: Author. http://www.rerf.or.jp/shared/ds02/index.html (accessed June 23, 2009).

Robinson, L. A. 2008. *Valuing mortality risk reductions in homeland security regulatory analyses.* Report to U.S. Customs and Border Protection, Department of Homeland Security. Cambridge, MA: Industrial Economics, Inc.

Rubinson, L., J. L. Hick, D. G. Hanfling, A. V. Devereaux, J. R. Dichter, M. D. Christian, D. Talmor, J. Medina, J. R. Curtis, and J. A. Geiling. 2008. Definitive care for the critically ill during a disaster: A framework for optimizing critical care surge capacity. From a Task Force for Mass Critical Care Summit Meeting, January 26-27, Chicago. *Chest* 133: 18S-31S. http://www.chestjournal.org/content/133/5_suppl/32S.full.pdf+html (accessed June 23, 2009).

Schreiber, M. 2005. PsySTART rapid mental health triage and incident management system. *The Dialogue* Summer:14-15. Quarterly technical assistance bulletin on disaster behavioral health of the Substance Abuse and Mental Health Services Administration, Rockville, MD. http://mentalhealth.samhsa.gov/dtac/dialogue/Summer2005.asp#six (accessed June 23, 2009).

Slovic, P., ed. 2001. *The perception of risk.* London, UK: Earthscan Publications.

Uraneck, K. 2008. *Planning for a nuclear incident: Tackling the "impossible."* Presentation at 2nd Emergency Management Summit, February 10, Washington, DC. http://www.ehcca.com/presentations/emsummit2/1_06.pdf (accessed June 23, 2009).

Vanderwagen, W. C. 2008. *Written testimony on HHS radiological/nuclear preparedness before the Senate Committee on Homeland Security and Governmental Affairs, June 26.* http://hsgac.senate.gov/public/_files/062608Vanderwagen.pdf (accessed June 23, 2009).

Veenema, T. G., B. Walden, N. Feinstein, and J. P. Williams. 2008. Factors affecting hospital-based nurses' willingness to respond to a radiation emergency. *Disaster Medicine and Public Health Preparedness* 2(4):224-229.

Ventura County. 2007. *Ventura County Nuclear Explosion Response Plan, Version 2.2.* Oxnard, CA: Ventura County Department of Public Health.

Waselenko, J. K., T. J. MacVittie, W. F. Blakely, N. Pesik, A. L. Wiley, W. E. Dickerson, H. Tsu, D. L. Confer, C. N. Coleman, T. Seed, P. Lowry, J. O. Armitage, and N. Dainiak. 2004. Medical management of the acute radiation syndrome: Recommendations of the Strategic National Stockpile Radiation Working Group. *Annals of Internal Medicine* 140(12):1037-1051. http://www.annals.org/cgi/reprint/140/12/1037.pdf (accessed June 23, 2009).

Weinstock, D. M., C. Case, Jr., J. L. Bader, N. J. Chao, C. N. Coleman, R. J. Hatchett, D. J. Weisdorf, and D. L. Confer. 2008. Radiologic and nuclear events: Contingency planning for hematologists/oncologists. *Blood* 111(12):5440-5445. http://bloodjournal.hematology library.org/cgi/reprint/111/12/5440 (accessed June 23, 2009).

Wray, R. J., S. M. Becker, N. Henderson, D. Glik, K. Jupka, S. Middleton, C. Henderson, A. Drury, and E. W. Mitchell. 2008. Communicating with the public about emerging health threats: Lessons from the Pre-Event Message Development Project. *American Journal of Public Health* 98(12):2214-2222. http://www.ajph.org/cgi/reprint/98/12/2214 (accessed June 23, 2009).

Appendix A

Workshop Agendas

> ASSESSING MEDICAL PREPAREDNESS TO RESPOND TO A
> TERRORIST NUCLEAR EVENT: WORKSHOP 1
> Committee on Medical Preparedness for a Terrorist Nuclear Event

PUBLIC AGENDA

Day 1
Thursday, June 26, 2008

Lecture Room
National Academy of Sciences
2101 Constitution Avenue, N.W.
Washington, DC

Workshop Objectives:

The purpose of the workshop is to assess the current level of medical preparedness for a nuclear detonation of up to 10 kilotons (kts) in Tier 1 Urban Area Security Initiative (UASI) cities (New York/New Jersey; National Capitol Region; Houston; Chicago; Los Angeles; and San Francisco/Bay Area). The specific objectives of the workshop are to

- review and summarize the overall emergency response activities and available health care capacity (including shelter, evacuation, decontamination, and medical infrastructure interdependencies) to treat the affected population;
- examine the capacity and identify gaps in the capability of the federal, state, and local authorities to deliver available medical countermeasures in a timely enough way to be effective;
- review and summarize available treatments for pertinent radiation illnesses, including the efficacy of medical countermeasures; and
- appraise the expected benefit of medical countermeasures, including those currently under development.

8:30 a.m.   Welcome, Introductions, and Overview of Workshop Purpose and Objectives

> GEORGES C. BENJAMIN, *Committee Chair*
> Executive Director
> American Public Health Association
>
> B. TILMAN JOLLY
> Office of Health Affairs
> Department of Homeland Security

SESSION 1

NUCLEAR ATTACK 101: HEALTH AND HEALTH SYSTEM IMPACTS OF AN IMPROVISED NUCLEAR DEVICE EXPLOSION

Session Objectives: Provide basic information on the scope of the emergency medical needs that would be created by the detonation of a 10-kt nuclear device in a major city, including primary and secondary blast and thermal effects and the effects of prompt nuclear radiation and radiation from fallout on inhabitants and emergency responders. The main focus will be on the acute injuries caused by the blast, thermal, and prompt radiation effects of the initial explosion and by acute radiation exposure from fallout during the first three days after the explosion (excluding other important but longer-term impacts, such as long-term radiation effects, environmental contamination, and displacement of residents from contaminated areas). The potential impacts of the explosion on local emergency response and health system capacities will also be described. At the end of the session, workshop participants will have a basic understanding of the medical situation faced by emergency responders during the first 3 days post-explosion, which in turn will be the basis for assessing current medical preparedness at the local, state, and federal levels.

9:00 a.m.   Session Overview and Objectives

               DANIEL F. FLYNN, *Session Moderator*
               Department of Radiation Oncology
               Caritas Holy Family Hospital and Medical Center
               Methuen, MA

9:05 a.m.   Health Effects of a 10-kt-Equivalent Nuclear Explosion on an Urban Population and Emergency Responders

               BROOKE BUDDEMEIER
               Radiation Safety Specialist
               Radiological and Nuclear Countermeasures
                  Division
               Global Security Principal Directorate
               Lawrence Livermore National Laboratory

9:35 a.m.   Health System Impacts of a 10-kt-Equivalent Nuclear Explosion on an Urban Area

               CHAM DALLAS
               Director, Institute for Health Management and
                  Mass Destruction Defense, University of Georgia
               Chair, Department of Health Policy and
                  Management, College of Public Health,
                  University of Georgia
               Department of Pharmaceutical & Biomedical
                  Sciences, College of Pharmacy, University of
                  Georgia
               Department of Emergency Medicine,
                  Medical College of Georgia

10:05 a.m.   Discussion led by

               Daniel F. Flynn, *Session Moderator*

10:35 a.m.   **BREAK**

SESSION 2

EMERGENCY MEDICAL CARE: STATE OF THE ART

Session Objective: Provide an overview of current approaches to medical response in the event of an improvised nuclear device (IND) explosion. The first presentation will cover the triage, decontamination, evacuation, and medical care of casualties from the immediate effects of a nuclear detonation (i.e., treatment of blast, thermal, and prompt radiation effects, including combined injuries). The second presentation will cover medical decision making and care of casualties from the delayed effects of a nuclear detonation (i.e., secondary triage and injuries from radioactive fallout).

10:45 a.m.   Session Overview and Objectives

> DONNA F. BARBISCH, *Session Moderator*
> President
> Global Deterrence Alternatives, LLC
> Washington, DC

10:50 a.m.   Urban Nuclear Detonation: Operational Conditions, Human Response and Casualty Management

> JOHN MERCIER
> Director of Military Medical Operations
> Armed Forces Radiobiology Research Institute

11:20 a.m.   Medical Decision Making and Care of Casualties from Delayed Effects of a Nuclear Detonation

> FRED A. METTLER, JR.
> Professor Emeritus
> Department of Radiology
> New Mexico Federal Regional Medical Center
> University of New Mexico

11:50 a.m.   Discussion led by

> DONNA F. BARBISCH, *Session Moderator*

12:20 p.m. **WORKING LUNCH IN THE LECTURE ROOM**
Committee, speakers, participants, and staff will briefly
recap the discussions from the morning sessions of the first
day of the workshop.

SESSION 3

RADIATION COUNTERMEASURES

Session Objective: Provide an overview of current medical countermeasures
for the acute effects of radiation exposure and of their efficacy as well as
an assessment of the expected benefit of medical countermeasures currently
under development.

1:30 p.m. Session Overview and Objectives

RICHARD J. HATCHETT, *Session Moderator*
Associate Director of Radiation Countermeasures
Research and Emergency Preparedness
National Institute of Allergy and Infectious Diseases

1:35 p.m. Efficacy and Expected Benefit of Currently Available
Radiation Countermeasures

ALBERT L. WILEY, JR.
Radiation Emergency Assistance Center/Training
Site and World Health Organization
Collaborating Center for Radiation Emergency
Assistance
Oak Ridge Associated Universities

2:05 p.m. Expected Benefit of Radiation Countermeasures Currently
Under Development

NELSON J. CHAO
Professor of Medicine and Immunology
Chief, Division of Cellular Therapy
Duke University Medical Center

2:35 p.m.   Distribution and Dispensing of Medical Countermeasures (i.e., How and When Will Countermeasures Get to Those Who Need Them?)

> CARMEN T. MAHER
> Policy Analyst
> Office of Counterterrorism and Emerging Threats
> Food and Drug Administration
>
> STEVEN A. ADAMS
> Deputy Director
> Division of Strategic National Stockpile
> Centers for Disease Control and Prevention

3:00 p.m.   Discussion led by

> RICHARD J. HATCHETT, *Session Moderator*

3:30 p.m.   **BREAK**

SESSION 4

PROTECTIVE ACTIONS AND INTERVENTIONS: PART I

Session Objective: Provide an overview of current policies and programs to protect first responders and medical personnel from radiation exposure.

3:45 p.m.   Session Overview and Objectives

> PAUL E. PEPE, *Session Moderator*
> Professor of Medicine, Surgery, Pediatrics, and Public Health and Riggs Family Chair in Emergency Medicine
> University of Texas Southwestern Medical Center at Dallas

3:50 p.m.   Radiation Protection Standards

> SARA D. DECAIR
> Health Physicist
> Center for Radiological Emergency Preparedness, Prevention, and Response
> Environmental Protection Agency

JOHN MACKINNEY
Deputy Director
Nuclear/Radiological/Chemical Threats and
    Science and Technology Policy, Office of Policy
    Development
Department of Homeland Security

JILL A. LIPOTI
Director
Division of Environmental Safety and Health
New Jersey Department of Environmental
    Protection

ERIC G. DAXON
Health Physicist
Battelle Memorial Institute–San Antonio Operations

4:40 p.m.   Discussion led by

PAUL E. PEPE, *Session Moderator*

5:10 p.m.   **ADJOURNMENT**

**ASSESSING MEDICAL PREPAREDNESS TO RESPOND TO A
TERRORIST NUCLEAR EVENT: WORKSHOP 1**
Committee on Medical Preparedness for a Terrorist Nuclear Event

---

PUBLIC AGENDA

Day 2
Friday, June 27, 2008

Auditorium
National Academy of Sciences
2101 Constitution Avenue, N.W.
Washington, DC

8:30 a.m.   Welcome, Introductions, and Overview of Workshop
Purpose and Objectives

GEORGES C. BENJAMIN, *Committee Chair*
Executive Director
American Public Health Association

SESSION 5

PROTECTIVE ACTIONS AND INTERVENTIONS: PART II

Session Objective: Provide overview of best population protection practices during an IND incident. Issues include risk communication, psychosocial factors, and readiness to implement interventions to reduce mental and physical impacts.

8:45 a.m.   Session Overview and Objectives

ROBERT J. URSANO, *Session Moderator*
Professor of Psychiatry and Neuroscience
Chairman, Department of Psychiatry
Uniformed Services University of the Health
    Sciences

8:50 a.m.   Behavioral and Risk Communication Issues, and
Intervention Strategies, in Nuclear Detonation Incidents

STEVEN M. BECKER
Associate Professor of Public Health
Vice Chair, Department of Environmental Health
    Sciences
Director, Disaster and Emergency Communication
    Research Unit
Director, Community Resilience and Disaster
    Management Program
University of Alabama at Birmingham

H. KEITH FLORIG
Senior Research Engineer
Department of Engineering and Public Policy
Carnegie Mellon University

ANN E. NORWOOD
Senior Associate
Center for Biosecurity
University of Pittsburgh Medical Center

DORI B. REISSMAN
Senior Medical Advisor
Office of the Director
National Institute for Occupational Safety and
Health

10:20 a.m.   BREAK

10:20 a.m.   Behavioral and Risk Communication Issues, and
Intervention Strategies, in Nuclear Detonation Incidents
(continued)

11:00 a.m.   Discussion led by

ROBERT J. URSANO, *Session Moderator*

SESSION 6

SUMMARY

11:30 a.m.   Summary of workshop discussions

JEROME M. HAUER
The Hauer Group

12:00 p.m.   Wrap-up and final thoughts

GEORGES C. BENJAMIN, *Committee Chair*

12:30 p.m.   ADJOURNMENT OF OPEN SESSION

ASSESSING MEDICAL PREPAREDNESS TO RESPOND TO A
TERRORIST NUCLEAR EVENT: WORKSHOP 2

Committee on Medical Preparedness for a Terrorist Nuclear Event

---

AGENDA

Day 1
Thursday, August 7, 2008

Auditorium
National Academy of Sciences
2101 Constitution Avenue, N.W.
Washington, DC

Workshop Objectives:

The purpose of the workshop is to assess the current level of medical preparedness for a nuclear detonation of up to 10 kts in Tier 1 Urban Area Security Initiative cities (New York/New Jersey; National Capitol Region; Houston; Chicago; Los Angeles; and San Francisco/Bay Area). The specific objectives of the workshop are to

- review and summarize the overall emergency response activities and available health care capacity (including shelter, evacuation, decontamination, and medical infrastructure interdependencies) to treat the affected population;
- examine the capacity and identify gaps in the capability of the federal, state, and local authorities to deliver available medical countermeasures in a timely enough way to be effective;
- review and summarize available treatments for pertinent radiation illnesses including the efficacy of medical countermeasures; and
- appraise the expected benefit of medical countermeasures, including those currently under development.

8:30 a.m.   Welcome, Introductions, and Overview of Workshop
              Purpose and Objectives

                    GEORGES C. BENJAMIN, *Committee Chair*
                    Executive Director
                    American Public Health Association

SESSION 1

CURRENT PREPAREDNESS FOR AN IMPROVISED NUCLEAR DEVICE, PART I: IMMEDIATE CASUALTIES

Session Objective: In response to the committee's statement of task, this session will explore the current level of medical preparedness for detonation of an IND of up to 10 kts in yield in a Tier 1 Urban Area Security Initiative area. Panels of local, state, and federal emergency response and medical personnel will review overall emergency response preparedness and capacity of the health care system to treat the population injured by the blast, thermal, and prompt radiation from an IND detonation, including the capacity of emergency medical services (EMS) to triage, treat, and transport the injured to treatment facilities and the capacity of the health care system to provide appropriate medical care to the numbers, types, and severities of likely injuries. The panels will address four aspects of emergency response preparedness: (1) the capacity of the emergency medical response to reach the injured and perform field triage and treatment, (2) the capacity to transport injured to area health care facilities, (3) the capacity of area health care facilities to evaluate and treat the likely numbers and types of injuries, and (4) the capacity to evacuate those who are seriously injured to appropriate health care facilities nationally.

8:55 a.m.   Session Overview and Objectives

GEORGE J. ANNAS, *Session Moderator*
Edward Utley Professor and Chair
Department of Health Law, Bioethics and Human
   Rights
Boston University School of Public Health

9:00 a.m.   **Panel 1.** Preparedness for emergency response to the detonation of a 10-kt IND (i.e., What capability is there to reach, triage, and treat those injured by the detonation safely?)

JOHN F. BROWN, San Francisco (San Francisco EMS
   Agency)
BROOKE BUDDEMEIER, Lawrence Livermore
National Laboratory

MICHAEL FITTON, New York (Fire Department of
New York)
KATHLEEN "CASS" KAUFMAN, Los Angeles
(Los Angeles County Department of Public
Health)
JOSEPH S. NEWTON, Chicago (Chicago Fire
Department)
RICHARD P. ZULEY, Chicago (Chicago Department
of Public Health)

10:00 a.m.   **Panel 2.** Preparedness to transport casualties to area treatment facilities (i.e., What capability is there to know
which treatment facilities are open, and what is the capacity to get them there?)

RICHARD L. ALCORTA, National Capital Region
(Maryland Institute for EMS Systems)
CRAIG DEATLEY, National Capital Region
(Washington Hospital Center, Washington, DC)
BRYAN HANLEY, Los Angeles (Los Angeles County
EMS Agency)
DOUGLAS HAVRON, Houston (Southeast Texas
Trauma Regional Advisory Council)
CARL E. LINDGREN, National Capital Region
(Arlington Fire Department, Virginia)

11:00 a.m.   **BREAK**

11:15 a.m.   **Panel 3.** Preparedness of the metropolitan area's medical
system to treat casualties from a 10-kt IND

JOSEPH A. BARBERA, Institute for Crisis, Disaster,
and Risk Management, George Washington
University
JOHN F. BROWN, San Francisco (San Francisco EMS
Agency)
PATRICIA HAWES, National Capital Region
(Suburban Hospital, Bethesda, Maryland)
NATHANIEL HUPERT, Weill Medical College of
Cornell University
AMY HIDEKO KAJI, Los Angeles (Harbor-UCLA
Medical Center)
KATHERINE URANECK, New York (New York City
Department of Health and Mental Hygiene)

12:15 p.m.   WORKING LUNCH TO CONTINUE PANEL
DISCUSSIONS

1:00 p.m.   **Panel 4.** Preparedness to evacuate serious casualties from
a 10-kt IND from area hospitals to appropriate treatment
facilities statewide and nationally

> JOSEPH A. BARBERA, George Washington University
> DAN HANFLING, National Capital Region
> (Inova Health System, Falls Church, Virginia)
> JEROME M. HAUER, The Hauer Group
> AASHISH SHAH, Houston (Texas Department of
> State Health Services)
> KATHERINE URANECK, New York (New York City
> Department of Health and Mental Hygiene)

2:00 p.m.   State of Preparedness for Immediate Casualties: An Open
Discussion by Committee Members and Audience

3:00 p.m.   **BREAK**

SESSION 2

CURRENTLY AVAILABLE MEDICAL RESOURCES

Session Objective: Discuss federal and state medical preparedness for an
IND event in a Tier 1 UASI area, the assets that will be available in such
an event, and the plans to use those assets.

3:15 p.m.   Session Overview and Objectives

> JUDITH A. MONROE, *Session Moderator*
> State Health Commissioner
> Indiana State Department of Health
> President, Association of State and Territorial
> Health Officials

3:20 p.m.   Department of Health and Human Services Response Assets and Plans in the Event of an IND Detonation

> ANN R. KNEBEL
> Office of the Assistant Secretary for Preparedness and Response
> Department of Health and Human Services

3:35 p.m.   Department of Energy Response Assets and Plans in the Event of an IND Detonation

> ALAN L. REMICK
> Office of Emergency Response
> National Nuclear Security Administration
> Department of Energy

3:50 p.m.   National Guard Response Assets and Plans in the Event of an IND Detonation

> COL. DANIEL BOCHICCHIO
> U.S. Army War College

4:05 p.m.   State Preparedness for an IND Event

> JAMES S. BLUMENSTOCK
> Association of State and Territorial Health Officials

4:20 p.m.   Discussion led by

> JUDITH A. MONROE, *Session Moderator*

5:20 p.m.   **ADJOURNMENT**

ASSESSING MEDICAL PREPAREDNESS TO RESPOND TO A
TERRORIST NUCLEAR EVENT: WORKSHOP 2

Committee on Medical Preparedness for a Terrorist Nuclear Event

AGENDA

Day 2
Friday, August 8, 2008

Auditorium
National Academy of Sciences
2101 Constitution Avenue, N.W.
Washington, DC

8:00 a.m.   Welcome, Introductions, and Overview of Workshop
              Purpose and Objectives

              GEORGES C. BENJAMIN, *Committee Chair*
              Executive Director
              American Public Health Association

SESSION 3

CURRENT PREPAREDNESS FOR AN IMPROVISED
NUCLEAR DEVICE, PART II:
PREVENTING AND TREATING FALLOUT CASUALTIES

Session Objective: Discuss the preparedness of Tier 1 UASI areas to manage the effects of the radiation fallout from a 10-kt IND and to identify,
mitigate, and manage long-term effects. Issues include effectiveness of risk
communication, short- and long-term mental health, efficacy of nonmedical protective actions such as sheltering in place and evacuation, and plans
and expectations for state and federal response resources to augment local
resources. This session will conclude with an assessment of what remains
to be done.

8:30 a.m.   Session Overview and Objectives

> COLLEEN CONWAY-WELCH, *Session Moderator*
> Nancy and Hilliard Travis Professor of Nursing
> Dean, Vanderbilt University School of Nursing

8:35 a.m.   **Panel 5.** Preparedness to mitigate, identify, and address fallout casualties and to manage long-term consequences

> THOMAS N. AHRENS, Los Angeles and San Francisco
> (California Department of Public Health)
> BROOKE BUDDEMEIER, Lawrence Livermore
> National Laboratory
> KATHLEEN "CASS" KAUFMAN, Los Angeles (Los
> Angeles County Department of Public Health)
> JEANINE PRUD'HOMME, New York (New York City
> Department of Health and Mental Hygiene)
> IRWIN REDLENER, Columbia University
> ADELA SALAME-ALFIE, New York (New York State
> Department of Health)
> REUBEN K. VARGHESE, National Capital Region
> (Arlington Public Health, Virginia)
> MICHAEL WELLING, National Capital Region
> (Virginia Department of Health)

10:30 a.m.   **BREAK**

10:45 a.m.   State of Preparedness for Fallout Casualties: An Open Discussion by Committee Members and Audience

---

SESSION 4

SUMMARY

11:30 a.m.   Wrap-up and final thoughts

> GEORGES C. BENJAMIN, *Committee Chair*
> Executive Director
> American Public Health Association

12:00 p.m.   **ADJOURN WORKSHOP**

Appendix B

Registered Workshop Attendees[*]

ASSESSING MEDICAL PREPAREDNESS TO RESPOND TO A
TERRORIST NUCLEAR EVENT: WORKSHOP 1

ISAF AL-NABULSI, National Council on Radiation Protection and
Measurements, Veterans' Advisory Board on Dose Reconstruction

RODELL ANDERSON, Defense Capabilities and Management Team,
Government Accountability Office, Washington, DC

TSVI ARANOFF, Office of the Assistant Secretary for Preparedness and
Response, Department of Health and Human Services

JUDITH BADER (Capt.), Office of the Assistant Secretary for
Preparedness and Response, Department of Health and Human
Services

TALI BAR-SHALOM, Office of Management and Budget, Executive
Office of the President

WILLIAM BELL, Institute for Health Management and Mass Destruction
Defense, University of Georgia

JESSICA BENJAMIN, National Institute of Allergy and Infectious
Diseases, National Institutes of Health

JOSH BERGMAN, Applied Research Associates, Inc., Arlington, VA

SAMUEL BIGGER, Nuclear National Security Administration,
Department of Energy

---

[*]This list includes the names and affiliations of the attendees who registered at the two work-shop events. It does not include the names of presenters indicated in the workshop agendas in Appendix A or committee members. Biographies of these individuals can be found in Appendix C and Appendix D, respectively.

CHERYL BITHER, U.S. Army Medical Materiel Agency, Federal Emergency Management Agency

WILLIAM BLAKELY, Scientific Research Department, Armed Forces Radiobiology Research Institute, Bethesda, MD

CHARLES BLUE (CAPT.), Office of Health Affairs, Department of Homeland Security

ARNOLD BOGIS, Belfer Center for Science and International Affairs, Harvard Kennedy School

LUCIANA BORIO, Center for Biosecurity of the University of Pittsburgh Medical Center, Baltimore, MD

JULIA BURR, Institute for Defense Analyses, Alexandria, VA

SANDRA BURRELL, Government Accountability Office, Washington, DC

DUANE CANEVA, Medical Preparedness Policy, White House Homeland Security Council

ELLEN CARLIN, Committee on Homeland Security, U.S. House of Representatives

CULLEN CASE, JR., National Marrow Donor Program, Radiation Injury Treatment Network, Minneapolis, MN

DAVID CASSATT, Division of Allergy, Immunology, and Transplantation/ National Institute of Allergy and Infectious Diseases, National Institutes of Health

RICK CHRISTENSEN, National Nuclear Security Administration, Department of Energy

ZACHARY COILE, *San Francisco Chronicle*

NORMAN COLEMAN, Office of the Assistant Secretary for Preparedness and Response, Department of Health and Human Services

THOMAS COTTON, JK Research Associates, Washington, DC

MIKE DAILY, private citizen

DANIEL DALTON, National Nuclear Security Administration, Department of Energy

WILLIAM DICKERSON (COL.), Red Cross, National Naval Medical Center, Bethesda, MD

MIKE FANELLI, Texas Christian University

AARON M. FIROVED, Homeland Security and Governmental Affairs Committee, U.S. Senate

DAVID FOX, Government Accountability Office, Washington, DC

ADAM FRANKEL, U.S. Strategies Corporation, Alexandria, VA

HARRY GEDNEY, National Park Service, National Mall and Memorial Parks, Washington, DC

MARCY GRACE, Scientific Research Department, Armed Forces Radiobiology Research Institute, Bethesda, MD

PATRICIA HAWES, Emergency Management, Suburban Hospital, Bethesda, MD

JACK HERRMANN, Preparedness Division, National Association of County and City Health Officials

MICHAEL HOPMEIER, Unconventional Concepts, Inc.

DAVID HOWELL, Pardee RAND Graduate School, RAND Corp, Arlington, VA

JOHN HOYLE, Disaster Operations and Recovery, Federal Emergency Management Agency National Emergency Training Center, Emmitsburg, MD

KOREY JACKSON (COL.), Nuclear Defense Policy, White House Homeland Security Council

KOSOKO JACKSON, National Institute for Occupational Safety and Health

ANN JAKUBOWSKI, Memorial Sloan-Kettering Cancer Center, New York

DAVID JARRETT, Office of the Secretary of Defense, Department of Defense

JOE KAMINSKI, Division of Allergy, Immunology, and Transplantation, National Institute of Allergy and Infectious Diseases, National Institutes of Health

DAVID KESTENBAUM, National Public Radio

WESLEY KIDDER, Government Relations, American Society for Therapeutic Radiology and Oncology

YAKOV KOGAN, Cleveland BioLabs, Inc., Buffalo, NY

MICHAEL LANDAUER, Armed Forces Radiobiology Research Institute, Bethesda, MD

ALEXANDRA LANDSBERG, U.S. Department of Homeland Security

WALTER LANGE, Nuclear Regulatory Commission

PATRICIA LILLIS-HEARNE, Armed Forces Radiobiology Research Institute, Bethesda, MD

BERT MAIDMENT, Division of Allergy, Immunology, and Transplantation, National Institute of Allergy and Infectious Diseases, National Institutes of Health

HANS MARK, University of Texas

RICHARD MARTIN, Government Relations, American Society for Therapeutic Radiology and Oncology

MICHAEL McCREERY, Medical Countermeasures Against Radiological Threats Program, University of Maryland School of Medicine, Baltimore

ANDREW MENER, National Center for Disaster Preparedness, Mailman School of Public Health, Columbia University

MARIA MORONI, Armed Forces Radiobiology Research Institute, Bethesda, MD

DAVID MORSE, Armed Forces Radiobiology Research Institute, Bethesda, MD

MICHAEL NOSKA (Capt.), Center for Devices and Radiological Health, Food and Drug Administration

CINDY NOTOBARTOLO, Safety/Security/ED Services, Suburban Hospital, Bethesda, MD

NATALIA OSSETROVA, Armed Forces Radiobiology Research Institute, Bethesda, MD

MICHAEL PETERS, Government Relations, American College of Radiology, Washington, DC

JOAN PFINSGRAFF, Health Intelligence, iJET International, Annapolis, MD

AMANDA POTTER, American Association of Physicists in Medicine, College Park, MD

DUDLEY RAINE, Applied Research Associates, Inc., Arlington, VA

IRWIN REDLENER, National Center for Disaster Preparedness, Mailman School of Public Health, Columbia University

GLEN REEVES, Radiation Effects, Northrop Grumman IT, Lorton, MD

DAVID SANDGREN, Armed Forces Radiobiology Research Institute, Bethesda, MD

D. MICHAEL SCHAEFFER, Science Applications International Corporation, McLean, VA

REGINA WATSON, Defense Threat Reduction Agency, Ft. Belvoir, VA

JOSEPH WEISS, Office of International Health Programs, Department of Energy, Germantown, MD

CINDY WELSH, Food and Drug Administration, Department of Health and Human Services

ROBERT WHITCOMB, Radiation Studies Branch, Centers for Disease Control and Prevention, Atlanta, GA

MARY WHITTAKER, Computer Science, George Washington University, Washington, DC

LINDA WILLIAMS, Central Arkansas Veterans Healthcare System, North Little Rock

EMILY WILSON, Government Relations, American Society for Therapeutic Radiology and Oncology

AIGUO WU, Reachback Medical Team, Defense Threat Reduction Agency, Ft. Belvoir, VA

WAYNE YOUNG, Biomedical Advanced Research and Development Authority, Department of Health and Human Services

ASSESSING MEDICAL PREPAREDNESS TO RESPOND TO A
TERRORIST NUCLEAR EVENT: WORKSHOP 2

STEVEN A. ADAMS, Division of Strategic National Stockpile, Centers
for Disease Control and Prevention, Atlanta, GA

RODELL ANDERSON, Defense Capabilities and Management Team,
Government Accountability Office, Washington, DC

JUDITH BADER (Capt.), Office of the Assistant Secretary for
Preparedness and Response, Department of Health and Human
Services

JONATHAN BAN, Office of the Assistant Secretary for Preparedness and
Response, Department of Health and Human Services

JESSICA BENJAMIN, National Institute of Allergy and Infectious
Diseases, National Institutes of Health

SAMUEL BIGGER, Office of Emergency Operations, Nuclear National
Security Administration, Department of Energy

ARNOLD BOGIS, Belfer Center for Science and International Affairs,
Harvard Kennedy School

DAVID CASSATT, Division of Allergy, Immunology, and Transplantation,
National Institute of Allergy and Infectious Diseases, National
Institutes of Health

RICK CHRISTENSEN, Emergency Operations, National Nuclear
Security Administration, Department of Energy

NORMAN COLEMAN, Office of the Assistant Secretary for
Preparedness and Response, Department of Health and Human
Services

SUSAN COLLER, Office of Preparedness and Emergency Operations,
Department of Health and Human Services

THOMAS COTTON, JK Research Associates, Washington, DC

DANIEL DALTON, Office of Emergency Management, National Nuclear
Security Administration, Department of Energy

SARA D. DeCAIR, Center for Radiological Emergency Preparedness,
Prevention, and Response, Environmental Protection Agency

ANDREA DiCARLO-COHEN, National Institute of Allergy and
Infectious Diseases, National Institutes of Health

WILLIAM DICKERSON (Col.), Radiation Oncology, National Naval
Medical Center, Bethesda, MD

RACHEL EISENSTEIN, Public Health Preparedness, National
Association of County and City Health Officials, Washington, DC

ANDREW GARRETT, National Center for Disaster Preparedness,
Mailman School of Public Health, Columbia University

MARCY GRACE, Chemical, Radiological and Nuclear Medical
Countermeasures, Project BioShield, Biomedical Advanced Research

and Development Authority, Department of Health and Human
Services

MICHAEL HOPMEIER, Unconventional Concepts, Inc., Mary Esther,
Florida

DAVID HOWELL, Pardee RAND Graduate School, RAND Corporation,
Arlington, VA

JOHN HOYLE, Disaster Operations and Recovery, Federal Emergency
Management Agency National Emergency Training Center,
Emmitsburg, MD

KOREY JACKSON (COL.), Nuclear Defense Policy, White House
Homeland Security Council

DAVID JARRETT, Office of the Secretary of Defense, Department of
Defense

JOSEPH KAMINSKI, National Institutes of Health

JONATHAN M. KRADEN, Committee on Homeland Security and
Government Affairs, U.S. Senate

GRAYDON LORD, National EMS Preparedness Initiative, Homeland
Security Policy Institute, George Washington University, Ashburn, VA

JOHN MacKINNEY, Nuclear/Radiological/Chemical Threats and Science
and Technology Policy, U.S. Department of Homeland Security

BERT MAIDMENT, Division of Allergy, Immunology, and
Transplantation, National Institute of Allergy and Infectious Diseases,
National Institutes of Health

DAVID MARCOZZI, Office of the Assistant Secretary for Preparedness
and Response, Department of Health and Human Services, and
White House Homeland Security Council

RICHARD MARTIN, Government Relations, American Society for
Therapeutic Radiology and Oncology

ANN E. NORWOOD, Center for Biosecurity of the University of
Pittsburgh Medical Center, Baltimore, MD

MICHAEL NOSKA (CAPT.), Center for Devices and Radiological Health,
Radiation Programs Branch, Food and Drug Administration

VICTOR OANCEA, Biomedical Advanced Research and Development
Authority/Science Applications International Corporation,
Department of Health and Human Services

GREGG PANE, National Healthcare Preparedness Programs, Office of
the Assistant Secretary for Preparedness and Response, Department
of Health and Human Services

MICHAEL PETERS, Government Relations, American College of
Radiology, Washington, DC

SAJEED POPAT, D.C. Homeland Security Emergency Management
Agency

AMANDA POTTER, American Association of Physicists in Medicine, College Park, MD

DUDLEY RAINE, Applied Research Associates, Inc., Arlington, VA

GLEN REEVES, Northrop Grumman Information Technology

THOMAS RUNYON, U.S. Army Center for Health Promotion and Preventive Medicine, Department of Defense, Aberdeen Proving Ground, MD

JAMES RUSH, Medical Logistics, JVR Health Readiness, Forest Hill, MD

REGINA WATSON, Reachback Medical Team, Defense Threat Reduction Agency, Ft. Belvoir, VA

ROBERT WHITCOMB, Radiation Studies Branch, Centers for Disease Control and Prevention, Atlanta, GA

MARY WHITTAKER, Computer Science, George Washington University, Washington, DC

DAVID WILMOT, The National Guard Bureau

WAYNE YOUNG, Biomedical Advanced Research and Development Authority, Department of Health and Human Services

Appendix C

Biographical Sketches of Workshop Speakers and Panelists

WORKSHOP SPEAKERS AND PANELISTS

Steven A. Adams, M.P.H., has served as the deputy director of the U.S. Strategic National Stockpile (SNS) Program located within the Department of Health and Human Services' (HHS') Centers for Disease Control and Prevention (CDC) from the time of its inception in 1999. As such, he has been intimately involved with the development and evolution of the national doctrine for response to public health crises and directly engaged with state and local authorities in the planning and implementation of the civilian medical response to large-scale public health emergencies. In addition to programmatic leadership, Mr. Adams has managed large-scale emergency responses and led CDC's rapid field response teams in the aftermath of events such as 9/11. He has served CDC in a variety of leadership roles for 20 years in contingency response programs as well as in public health efforts as varied as human immunodeficiency virus (HIV) field research and radiological dose reconstruction related to Cold War–era nuclear weapons production. Mr. Adams earned an M.P.H. from the University of North Carolina at Chapel Hill.

Thomas N. Ahrens, Pharm.D., currently serves as chief of Emergency Pharmaceutical Services for the California Department of Public Health (CDPH). He has served as the California SNS Coordinator since January 2001. Dr. Ahrens coordinates and supervises all CDPH programs on emergency response and recovery activities and services related to the SNS (including the Chempack Project, the Cities Readiness Initiative, selection of and purchase of pharmaceuticals for the Hospital Preparedness Program and the state's antiviral cache for pandemic preparedness) and all CDPH's emergency plans pertaining to the requesting of medical supplies and pharmaceuticals in response to planning needs and emergency response. He has been directly involved in various emergency response activations of the State Emergency Operations Center and has served as a Public Health Agency representative and a Public Health Branch coordinator. In addition, Dr. Ahrens has served as the director of the CDPH Joint Emergency Operations Center during emergency response activations and as warehouse director during functional exercises involving the receipt and distribution of the SNS. His background includes working as a pharmacist, with 29 years experience with the California departments of health services, public health, and mental health, in addition to private hospital and retail pharmacy services. He received his doctor of pharmacy degree from the University of Southern California.

Richard L. Alcorta, M.D., FACEP, is a board-certified emergency medicine physician. He started his EMS career as an emergency medical technician–ambulance and went on to become a paramedic in California. While performing as an EMT-P in Imperial County, California, he also performed as a sworn sheriff reserve. He received his B.S. degree at San Diego State University. In 1983 he graduated from Howard University School of Medicine and was inducted into Alpha Omega Alpha (Honor Medical Society). He completed his emergency medicine residency at Harbor-University of California at Los Angeles (UCLA) Medical Center, and in 1986 he started as a faculty member of the emergency department at Johns Hopkins Medical Center. He has practiced emergency medicine at Suburban Hospital Shock Trauma Center since 1987. From 1992 to 1994 he was the state EMS director for Maryland, and in 1995 he was appointed the state EMS medical director at the Maryland Institute for Emergency Medical Services Systems. He has developed and delivered numerous presentations on chemical, biological, radiological, and traumatic (including blast) injures as well as on incident management to EMS, nurses, and physicians. He was the state medical director for the Chemical Stockpile Emergency Preparedness Program (CSEPP) during the neutralization of 1,600 tons of mustard chemical warfare agent in Maryland as well as a medical advisor to the U.S. Secret Service. Dr. Alcorta has spoken as a subject matter expert at National CSEPP, B.A.T.T.L.E. FBI, and National Disaster Medical System conferences.

Joseph A. Barbera, M.D., is codirector of the George Washington University Institute for Crisis, Disaster, and Risk Management and has blended clinical practice, academics, research, preparedness, and emergency response activities throughout his professional career. He is associate professor of engineering management and clinical associate professor of emergency medicine at George Washington University. Dr. Barbera created and teaches masters- and doctoral-level academic courses in emergency management and has completed multiple applied research projects focusing on health and medical systems in emergency response. He directed emergency management activi- ties at teaching hospitals in New York (Bronx Municipal Hospital Center) and Washington, DC (George Washington University Hospital), and he has provided emergency management consultation and training for a wide vari- ety of health care organizations and federal and state agencies. Dr. Barbera coordinated implementation of one of the first hospital mass patient decon- tamination and treatment facilities and chaired the establishment of a com- prehensive hospital mutual aid system in Washington, DC, well before the 9/11 generated attention in this area. He has enjoyed a 2-decade career as an emergency responder to major disasters for the U.S. government and others. Experiences include scene response to hurricanes (2005 Hurricanes Katrina and Wilma and others), mine disasters, earthquakes (Baguio City, Philippines; Northridge, California; and Tou-Liu, Taiwan), mass terrorism (the Oklahoma City bombing and the 9/11 Pentagon and World Trade Center attack sites), biological terrorism (anthrax, 2001), and tsunami (Banda Aceh, Indonesia). Dr. Barbera has authored numerous scientific and technical papers related to medical and public health emergency manage- ment. He earned his M.D. from the University of Pittsburgh School of Medi- cine and completed residency training in both family practice (University of Connecticut) and emergency medicine (Albert Einstein College of Medicine), and he maintains board certification in emergency medicine.

Steven M. Becker, Ph.D., is associate professor of public health and vice chair of the Department of Environmental Health Sciences at the University of Alabama at Birmingham. Dr. Becker has nearly two decades of experience dealing with the public health, emergency planning, community response, and risk communication aspects of incidents involving invisible toxic agents. He is one of only a small number of U.S. researchers to have carried out extensive overseas fieldwork related to all three major types of invisible agents: chemicals, infectious disease, and radiation. This includes fieldwork during a major chemical accident in Great Britain; onsite work during the 1999 nuclear accident in Tokaimura, Japan; follow-up work in Ukraine and Belarus related to the Chernobyl nuclear disaster; and fieldwork during the 2001 foot-and-mouth disease outbreak in the United Kingdom. Dr. Becker served as principal investigator for the radiological/nuclear risk communi- cation component of the Pre-Event Message Development Project, a major CDC-funded study to improve emergency communication during terrorism incidents. The multiyear, multisite project identified key concerns and infor- mation needs for the general public, first responders, hospital emergency department personnel, and the public health workforce. The project also provided the most extensive research to date on the public information aspects of improvised nuclear device (IND) scenarios. In 2005 Dr. Becker was elected to the National Council on Radiation Protection and Measurements, where he also serves as a member of the Advisory Panel on Public Policy and PAC 3 (Nuclear and Radiological Safety and Security). In addition, Dr. Becker has served on several national policy panels dealing with CBRNE terrorism and is a coauthor of the landmark NCRP 138 report, *Management of Terrorist Incidents Involving Radioactive Material.*

James S. Blumenstock became chief program officer, public health practice, for the Association of State and Territorial Health Officials (ASTHO) in June 2007. His portfolio includes the state public health practice program areas of infectious and emerging diseases, immunization, environmental health, injury prevention, and public health preparedness and security, including pandemic influenza preparedness. He also serves as a member of the association's executive management team responsible for enterprise-wide strategic planning, administrative services, member support, and public health advocacy. Prior to his arrival at ASTHO on November 1, 2005, Mr. Blumenstock was the deputy commissioner of health for the New Jersey Department of Health and Senior Services, from which he retired after almost 32 years of career public health service. In this capacity, he had executive oversight responsibilities for a department branch with more than 650 staff members and an operating budget of approximately $125 million. The branch comprised the Division of Public Health and Environmental Laboratories; the Division of Epidemiology, Occupational, and Environmental Health; the Division of Local Health Practice and Regional Systems Development; the Division of Health Emergency Preparedness and Response; and the Office of Animal Welfare. During his tenure Mr. Blumenstock also represented the department on a number of boards, councils, and commissions, including the New Jersey Domestic Security Preparedness Task Force. He received the ASTHO 2004 Noble J. Swearingen Award for excellence in public health administration and the Dennis J. Sullivan award, the highest honor bestowed by the New Jersey Public Health Association, for dedicated and outstanding service and contribution to the cause of public health. He is also a Year 14 scholar of the Public Health Leadership Institute, and he held an elected office serving his community for 12 years. Mr. Blumenstock received his B.S. in environmental science from Rutgers University in 1973 and his M.A. in health sciences administration from Jersey City State College in 1977.

Daniel J. Bochicchio, M.D., FCCP, a decorated combat surgeon, currently serves as deputy chief surgeon on the Joint Staff of the National Guard Bureau in Arlington, Virginia. For the Office of the Surgeon he addresses medical issues related to domestic disaster preparedness and the development and implementation of policies to ensure smooth integration of National Guard medical assets into civilian disaster response plans. Colonel Bochicchio's role is to establish and mature strategic relationships with key Department of Defense (DoD) and federal civilian interagency partners to promote integration and unity of effort as required by the National Response Framework. In 2005 Colonel Bochicchio was the Battalion Surgeon for Task Force 1-172 (Armored) Marine Division in Iraq, where he was responsible for the coordination and delivery of emergency and routine medical care to soldiers and Marines during combat operations in Al-Anbar Province, Iraq. From 2004 to 2005 he was responsible for planning and developing the National Guard domestic chemical, biological, radiological, nuclear, or explosive (CBRNE) medical response as chief of Domestic Medical Operations for the National Guard Bureau. He was tasked with design and implementation of medical aspects of the National Guard CBRNE Enhanced Response Force Package teams and Weapon of Mass Destruction (WMD) Civil Support Teams. Colonel Bochicchio's previous assignments have included chief of the Division Medical Operations Center, Headquarters, Division Support Command, 29th Infantry Division and commander of Company C, 229th Support Battalion, 29th Infantry Division. He is board certified in anesthesiology and critical care medicine and is a former faculty member of the University of Maryland School of Medicine.

John F. Brown, M.D., M.P.A., has served as the medical director for the San Francisco EMS Agency, Department of Public Health, since 1996. In his current position he has been responsible for the development and implementation of local policies, procedures, and protocols for the pre-hospital emergency responders for the public safety agencies and private ambulance providers in San Francisco. He serves as the medical health operations area coordinator in the city's disaster response structure, and he has been medical advisor for the local Metropolitan Medical Response System program. He serves as a medical officer for the Disaster Medical Assistance Team CA-6 and is an assistant clinical professor in emergency medicine working at San Francisco General Hospital. Prior to his current position Dr. Brown served as the U.S. Navy Surgeon General's Advisor for EMS and worked at the San Diego Naval Medical Center after the completion of his residency in emergency medicine there. He performed a postdoctoral fellowship in emergency medical services and earned an M.P.A. at the University of Arizona. His M.D. is from the University of Connecticut.

Brooke Buddemeier, CHP, M.S., works for the Global Security Directorate of the Lawrence Livermore National Laboratory supporting risk and consequence management activities. He recently completed a 3.5-year assignment with the Department of Homeland Security as the weapons of mass destruction emergency response and consequence management program manager for the Science and Technology Directorate's emergency preparedness and response portfolio. He supported the Federal Emergency Management Agency and the Homeland Security Operations Center as a radiological emergency response subject matter expert. He also facilitated the department's research, development, test, and evaluation process to improve emergency response through better capabilities, protocols, and standards. He is a certified health physicist who received his M.S. in radiological health physics from San Jose State University and his B.S. in nuclear engineering from the University of California, Santa Barbara.

Nelson J. Chao, M.D., M.B.A., is professor of medicine and immunology and the chief of the Division of Cellular Therapy/Bone Marrow Transplant at Duke University. He received his undergraduate degree from Harvard University, his M.D. from Yale University, and his postgraduate training at Stanford University. He then joined the faculty at Stanford University. He was the associate director of Stem Cell Transplantation at Stanford University prior to moving to Duke University in 1996 to be the program director of the Bone Marrow Transplantation Program. The program became a division within the Department of Medicine in 2000 and was renamed the Division of Cellular Therapy/BMT. Dr. Chao is also the codirector of the Clinical Stem Cell Transplantation Laboratory, and he continues to direct his own research laboratory focused on understanding and preventing graft-versus-host disease and improving immune reconstitution. He also directs the clinical research within the division. He obtained his M.B.A. from the Fuqua School of Business at Duke University in 2000. He is the author of approximately 200 peer-reviewed papers, book chapters, and 1 book. He is also a cofounder of Aldagen, a start-up biotechnology company in Research Triangle Park.

Cham Dallas, M.S., Ph.D., is professor and director of the Institute for Health Management and Mass Destruction Defense (IHMD) at the University of Georgia, interim director of the Department of Health Policy and Management at the College of Public Health, and a member of the Department of Emergency Medicine at the Medical College of Georgia (MCG). He received his M.S. and Ph.D. in toxicology from the University of Texas (UT) School of Public Health at Houston. For 7 years Dr. Dallas was the director of one of the largest university toxicology programs in the country, with 50 professors, at the University of Georgia. For 5 years he was the director of the Center for Mass Destruction Defense, a CDC Center for Public Health Preparedness dealing with mass casualty management. Dr. Dallas's institute has established a nationally successful collaboration with the American Medical Association (AMA), MCG, and UT for the development of the National Disaster Life Support (NDLS) family of courses. NDLS has been accepted as a national standard for WMDs training by the AMA and has been taught in 45 states to more than 60,000 health care personnel. Dr. Dallas and IHMD staff are currently conducting mass casualty evaluation exercises for Georgia hospitals as well as devising evacuation planning for special-needs populations. He has been the recipient of several teaching awards, including a university-wide award. He has written scores of research papers for the scientific community and educational articles for the public on the toxic components of WMDs. Dr. Dallas led a series of scientific expeditions to the most highly contaminated areas around Chernobyl and conducted research and teaching efforts there for more than 10 years, including at more than 40 institutions overseas. He has testified before the U.S. House and Senate Homeland Security hearings and at the United Nations three times on the topic of nuclear war medical response.

Eric G. Daxon (Colonel-Retired, U.S. Army), Ph.D., CHP, is currently a senior research scientist with Battelle Memorial Institute. His current work centers on policy, doctrine, and plans for radiological or nuclear events for DoD clients. His current work at Battelle and the past 15 years of his 30-year military career have focused on the integration of radiation risk into decision making for the full range of military deployments. As the army's medical lead for issues related to the use of depleted uranium munitions in combat, Dr. Daxon dealt directly with the issue of radiation risks and the risks of radiation exposure mitigation in emergency environments. Prior assignments include director of the Proponency Office for Preventive Medicine at the U.S. Army Center for Health Promotion and Preventive Medicine and the chair of the Radiation Biophysics Department at the Armed Forces Radiobiology Research Institute. Dr. Daxon has a Ph.D. in radiological hygiene from the University of Pittsburgh, an M.S. in nuclear engineering from the Massachusetts Institute of Technology, and a B.S. in engineering from the United States Military Academy at West Point.

Craig DeAtley, PA-C., is currently the director of the Institute for Public Health Emergency Readiness at Washington Hospital Center, the District of Columbia's largest hospital. Prior to taking this position he was an associate professor of emergency medicine at George Washington University, where he worked full-time for 28 years before leaving to start the institute. He also works as a physician assistant at Fairfax Hospital, a level 1 trauma center in Northern Virginia. In addition to being a physician assistant, he has been a volunteer paramedic with the Fairfax County Fire and Rescue Department since 1972 and a member of their Urban Search and Rescue Team since 1991. He currently serves as the team's medical team coordinator. Mr. DeAtley also serves as the assistant medical director for the Fairfax County Police Department. Those positions involve working with the special operations personnel (special weapons and tactics, civil disturbance, marine patrol, and helicopter operations) in those agencies. He has particular interest in hazardous material and WMD planning and response, and he was a founding member of NMRS-DC-1, the nation's first U.S. Public Health Service trained-and-equipped civilian nuclear, biological, and chemical incident response team. For the past 11 years he has been working as a consultant on projects related to DoD/Department of Justice WMD Domestic Preparedness Programs and on a variety of HHS/CDC Public Health Department projects regarding preparedness and response. Each of these projects has led to him working with police, fire, EMS, hospitals, emergency management, and mental health and public health personnel to develop and exercise their hazardous material/chemical-biological response plans. Mr. DeAtley also worked for the HHS Office of Emergency Preparedness in developing and facilitating a new Public Health Emergency Practicum Program for medical, emergency management, public health, and public safety personnel. His publications include recently serving as editor and contributing author for *Jane's Mass Casualty Handbook Pre-Hospital Care-Emergency Preparedness and Response*. He served as the project manager to assist Arlington County, Virginia, in writing and exercising the Isolation and Quarantine Annex to its Emergency Operations Plan. More recently he served as the comanager of the HEICS IV project done on behalf of the California EMS. This project led to the recent release of the new Hospital Incident Command System. In addition, the project personnel also provided feedback to the National Incident Management System Integration Center on the system's compliance activities for health care organizations.

Sara D. DeCair, B.S., has been a health physicist with the Office of Radiation and Indoor Air at the Environmental Protection Agency (EPA) since 2003. She works on policy, planning, training, and outreach for EPA's radiological emergency preparedness and response program. She is the project and technical lead for revising the Protective Action Guides and is especially interested in emergency worker dose limits and turnback levels. She previously worked for 7 years with the State of Michigan's Department of Environmental Quality. Three of those years were spent in nuclear power plant emergency planning, and before that she was an inspector of radioactive materials registrants and a radiation incident responder. She is currently the affiliates director of the Baltimore-Washington chapter of the Health Physics Society.

Michael Fitton has served the City of New York as a paramedic for the past 24 years. He began his career in pre-hospital care receiving and dispatching 911 calls throughout the city. His years as a paramedic in the Bronx brought his future career goals into focus. He earned instructor certification and taught both basic life support and advanced life support programs. He went on through the ranks of lieutenant, captain, and deputy chief. In these years Chief Fitton was the commanding officer at EMS stations, a city-wide dispatch supervisor at the Fire Department of New York's (FDNY's) Emergency Medical Dispatch Center, has served as a deputy chief citywide, and currently is the division commander of the borough of the Bronx. He was selected to participate in the FDNY and U.S. Military Academy's Joint Program for Combating Terrorism. Chief Fitton completed an intensive program at the Fire Officers Management Institute, a part of the Columbia University Graduate School Executive Development Program. He is currently pursuing a professional studies degree in emergency management at Empire State College/State University of New York.

H. Keith Florig, Ph.D., is senior research engineer in the Department of Engineering and Public Policy at Carnegie Mellon University, where he conducts research on public policy and communications issues involving health, safety, environment, and security risks. His work on the management and communication of radiation risks has been published in *Science, Health Physics, Risk Analysis,* and other journals. Dr. Florig has served on committees addressing radiation risks at both the National Council on Radiation Protection and Measurements and the National Academy of Sciences. In recognition of his work on public involvement in radiation protection, he was selected to deliver the 2004 G. William Morgan Lecture of the Health Physics Society. Dr. Florig holds degrees in engineering and public policy (Ph.D.), nuclear science and engineering (M.S.), instrumentation (M.S.), and physics (B.S.), all from Carnegie Mellon. Before joining the Carnegie Mellon faculty in 1996, he worked for 6 years in Washington, DC, at the U.S. Arms Control and Disarmament Agency and at Resources for the Future.

Dan Hanfling, M.D., is the director of Emergency Management and Disaster Medicine for the Inova Health System in Falls Church, Virginia. He is also the state medical director for PHI Air Medical Group-Virginia, the largest private rotor-wing air medevac service in the Commonwealth of Virginia. He serves as a medical team manager for Virginia Task Force 1, a Federal Emergency Management Agency (FEMA)- and U.S. Agency for International Development-sanctioned international urban search-and-rescue team, and he has been involved in the response to international and domestic disaster events, including the response to the Pentagon attack in September 2001 and the response to Hurricanes Rita and Katrina in 2005. Dr. Hanfling was intimately involved in the response to the anthrax bioterror mailings in the fall of 2001, when two cases of inhalational anthrax were successfully diagnosed at Inova Fairfax Hospital. He was a founding member and cochairman of the Northern Virginia Emergency Response Coalition and a founding member of the Northern Virginia Hospital Alliance. He has been appointed to the Virginia Secure Initiative Health and Medical Subpanel, the Virginia Department of Health Emergency Preparedness and Response Advisory Committee, and the Virginia Health and Hospitals Association Hospital Emergency Management Committee. Dr. Hanfling has testified before Congress on the issues of health care emergency management and disaster response. He lectures nationally and internationally on pre-hospital, hospital, and disaster-related subjects, and has coauthored numerous peer-reviewed articles on the subject of health care facility disaster preparedness. He received an A.B. in political science from Duke University and an M.D. from Brown University. He completed an internship in internal medicine at Miriam Hospital in Providence, Rhode Island, and an emergency medicine residency at George Washington/Georgetown University hospitals. He is a clinical professor of emergency medicine at George Washington University and an adjunct distinguished senior fellow at the George Mason University School of Public Policy.

Bryan Hanley is the regional disaster medical and health specialist representing the State of California Governor's Office of Emergency Services (OES) Mutual Aid Region One. OES Region One is home to nearly 14 million people living within Los Angeles, Orange, Ventura, Santa Barbara, and San Luis Obispo counties. Region One is a Tier 1 Urban Area Security Initiative area. Mr. Hanley is employed by the County of Los Angeles Emergency Medical Services Agency under contract with the State of California EMS Authority and California Department of Public Health. He works closely with county-level EMS agencies and public health departments in preparing their hospitals, fire service, EMS, law enforcement, and other medical and health partners to facilitate a coordinated response to natural or manmade disasters. Mr. Hanley also assists state agencies by facilitating integration of state priorities and projects into the local plans and efforts. During actual responses he coordinates information flow, requests for mutual aid, and reception of assistance into a disaster area as the director of the Medical and Health Branch of the Regional Emergency Operations Center (EOC). He serves as a member of various advisory groups locally and at the state level. Mr. Hanley has coordinated major response activities in his career, both at the field command level and within the command policy group in an EOC. He is a command staff member of the National Disaster Medical Assistance Team, California-1, based in Orange County. He has spent more than

20 years in emergency management and is a trained and licensed paramedic, a former firefighter, and a hazardous materials technician. His educational background includes advanced degrees in health science and criminal justice-law enforcement. He has received training at the National Fire Academy and FEMA's Emergency Management Institute in Emmitsburg, Maryland. He has had the opportunity to teach at the university and community college level, and he lectures throughout the nation and internationally on various emergency management and terrorist threat topics.

Jerome M. Hauer, M.P.H., one of the nation's best-known names in emergency management and health and medical response to disasters, is now the chief executive officer of the Hauer Group. He served as the first assistant secretary (acting) of the Office of Public Health Emergency Preparedness at HHS and was responsible for coordinating the country's medical and public health preparedness in response to emergencies, including acts of biological, chemical, and nuclear terrorism. Before that Mr. Hauer was New York City's first director of the Mayor's Office of Emergency Management and was charged with coordinating the city's planning for and response to natural and manmade events, including acts of terrorism. Prior to that he served as the executive director of the State of Indiana's Emergency Management Agency as well as its Department of Fire and Buildings. He was on the Congressional Fire Caucus's Urban Search and Rescue Advisory Committee as well as the National Institute for Urban Search and Rescue Advisory Council. Mr. Hauer served on the Institute of Medicine's (IOM's) Committee to Evaluate R&D Needs for Improved Civilian Medical Response to Chemical or Biological Terrorism Incidents, as consulting fellow at the Potomac Institute for Policy Studies' Center for Emerging Threat and Opportunities and at the Board of Visitors of the National Interagency Civil-Military Institute, and as an advisor to the U.S. Capitol Police and the U.S. Marine Corps' Chemical-Biological Incident Response Force. He served on the faculty of the Northeastern University Paramedic Program, and he codirected the first two postgraduate courses in trauma management at the Longwood Area Trauma Center of the Harvard Medical School. Mr. Hauer was a captain in the U.S. Army Reserve attached to the Walter Reed Army Institute of Research in Washington, DC. He has an M.P.H. from the Johns Hopkins School of Public Health and a bachelor's degree from New York University.

Douglas Havron, RN, B.S.N., M.S., CEN, CEM, is the administrative director for the Southeast Texas Trauma Regional Advisory Council and the Regional Hospital Preparedness Council. His responsibilities include the administrative leadership of the Hospital Preparedness Program for the Houston Metro area and surrounding counties. His experience includes

EMS, inner-city Level 1 trauma center management, hospital administration, and regional hospital preparedness leadership. He has more than 15 years of experience in disaster preparedness and response, and he served as one of Houston's medical operations chiefs for the Catastrophic Medical Operations Center during Hurricanes Katrina and Rita. He has a B.S.N. from the University of Texas–El Paso and an M.S. in emergency management from Touro University.

Patricia Hawes, RN, B.S.N., COHN, is the emergency manager for Suburban Hospital in Bethesda, Maryland, where she has helped lead the hospital to be named one of the top five most highly prepared trauma hospitals in the nation by the National Foundation for Trauma Care in conjunction with CDC. She is on the leadership board of the Bethesda Hospital's Emergency Preparedness Partnership, which is composed of the National Institutes of Health Clinical Center, the National Naval Medical Center, the National Library of Medicine, and Suburban Hospital. Ms. Hawes is the vice chair of the National Capital Region-Health and Medical Programmatic workgroup, where she represents the interests of Maryland hospitals. Ms. Hawes was also a contributing author of the National Capital Regional Surge Plan. She designs and participates in a yearly regional collaborative multiagency exercise that tests hospital surge preparedness. Ms. Hawes is a registered nurse with more than 20 years experience in trauma care and cardiothoracic intensive care and is certified in occupational health, having obtained her B.S.N. from Jacksonville University.

Nathaniel Hupert, M.D., M.P.H., is an associate professor of public health at Cornell University's Weill Medical College, an associate attending physician at New York-Presbyterian Hospital, and the director of the new Preparedness Modeling Initiative for CDC. Since 2000 he has led a number of federally funded projects to develop improved tools and logistics for mass prophylaxis, bioterrorism response, and health system preparedness for surge capacity. His research team's models are available on the websites of HHS and the American Hospital Association, and they are used by states across the United States for preparedness planning. One of three academic researchers to serve on the Anthrax Modeling Working Group of the HHS Secretary's Council on Public Health Emergency Preparedness, he has lectured and given satellite and web broadcasts for the Agency for Healthcare Research and Quality and CDC on mass prophylaxis and the physician's role in bioterrorism response. Dr. Hupert is codirector of Cornell's Institute for Disease and Disaster Preparedness, whose mission is to advance the field of computational public health by applying engineering approaches to a range of public health response logistics problems ranging from U.S.

emergency preparedness to scale-up of HIV/acquired immune deficiency syndrome treatment in sub-Saharan Africa.

Amy Hideko Kaji, M.D., Ph.D., is board certified in emergency medicine and acts as the medical director for the Harbor-UCLA South Bay Disaster Resource Center. She performed a disaster medicine and research fellowship at the UCLA School of Public Health, where she obtained both an M.P.H. and a Ph.D. in epidemiology. The focus of her dissertation was the assessment of hospital disaster preparedness and surge capacity in Los Angeles County. As such, she is knowledgeable about the management of mass casualty incidents and disaster response. As the medical director of 1 of 13 regional centers of excellence in disaster preparedness in Los Angeles County, she is actively engaged in coordinating disaster drills and classes as well as in stockpiling pharmaceuticals and supplies. She is also an assistant clinical professor of medicine in the Department of Emergency Medicine at the David Geffen School of Medicine at UCLA.

Ann R. Knebel (Captain, U.S. Public Health Service), RN, D.N.Sc., FAAN, is a registered nurse with a D.N.Sc. in pulmonary critical care. For the past 16 years she has served as an officer in the Public Health Service Commissioned Corps. Currently she is deputy director for preparedness planning with HHS in the Office of the Assistant Secretary for Preparedness and Response (ASPR). In this capacity, she is responsible for the development of programs to enhance preparedness integration across the local/state/regional and federal tiers of response. In the 6 years Dr. Knebel has worked for ASPR (formerly the Office of the Assistant Secretary for Public Health and Emergency Preparedness [OPHEP]), she has been instrumental in advancing various preparedness planning and surge capacity initiatives. Highlights include assisting the Greek Ministry of Health to prepare for the 2004 Summer Olympics and a 9-month detail with the New York City Office of Emergency Management to develop bioterrorism plans. During the response to the 2005 and 2008 hurricane seasons, Dr. Knebel worked as the plans section chief on the HHS Emergency Management Team, helping to plan the federal public health and medical response and recovery. Prior to joining ASPR, Dr. Knebel served in both the intramural and extramural programs at the National Institutes of Health. She is a fellow of the American Academy of Nursing.

Kathleen "Cass" Kaufman has been the director of the Los Angeles County Department of Public Health's radiation management program since 1990. Radiation management staff inspect all users of X-ray machines or radioactive materials to ensure compliance with California and federal laws and regulations, and they respond to radiation emergencies. Los Angeles County has been proactive in preparing to respond to a deliberate radiation event by providing training to fire departments, hospitals, and law enforcement and by acquiring specialized equipment to detect, assess, and respond to an event. In addition to programmatic leadership, Ms. Kaufman has direct experience in responding to radiation emergencies. Ms. Kaufman has served on many national committees and is on the Conference of Radiation Control Program Directors' Committee that wrote the *Handbook for Responding to a Radiological Dispersal Device.* She currently serves on the National Council on Radiation Protection committee that is writing a report to address key decisions that decision makers will need to make after a radiologic or nuclear event. Ms. Kaufman has a degree in radiological sciences from George Washington University in Washington, DC, and has taken numerous courses and participated in many exercises over the course of her career.

Carl E. Lindgren, NREMT-P, is a 28-year veteran of the Arlington County Fire Department in Virginia. He currently holds the rank of fire/EMS battalion chief with overall responsibility for EMS in North Arlington. Mr. Lindgren was part of the inaugural National Medical Response Team (NMRT) that later became the DC-NMRT. The majority of Mr. Lindgren's career was spent as a field EMS supervisor. During the 9/11 attack of the Pentagon (located in Arlington), Mr. Lindgren served as the treatment unit leader the day of the attack. After 9/11, Mr. Lindgren was assigned to be one of two operations training officers with a strong focus on EMS during a WMD event. His next assignment, in 2002, was to the county's newly expanded Office of Emergency Management. He was responsible for instructing county staff on the new emergency operations plan, along with responsibility for the county's Homeland Security Exercise and Evaluation Program. Participants included the Pentagon and United States Northern Command as well as the county's partners across the National Capital Region, with a focus on exercising, developing, and evaluating the region's capabilities. He was part of two Emergency Management Assistance Compact EOC deployments, one to Hurricane Charlie in Charlotte, Florida, and the second as the first EOC team to assemble and begin EOC operations in the city of New Orleans after Hurricane Katrina, for which he served as the Emergency Services Branch director. Mr. Lindgren has spoken on EMS, WMDs, public health, and emergency management across the globe. He received his AAS in emergency medicine in 1980 from Northern Virginia Community College as one of the early nationally registered paramedics in the state of Virginia.

Jill A. Lipoti, Ph.D., received her Ph.D. in environmental science from Rutgers University. She is the director of the Division of Environmental Safety and Health in the New Jersey Department of Environmental Protection. She has responsibility for radiation protection, chemical release prevention, lab certification and quality assurance, pollution prevention, and right to know. Dr. Lipoti served as a member of the board of directors and as chairperson for the Conference of Radiation Control Program Directors (CRCPD). In 2000 she received the Gerald S. Parker Award of Merit, CRCPD's highest award. She served as chair of the Radiation Advisory Committee of the Environmental Protection Agency's (EPA's) Science Advisory Board (SAB) and serves on its executive committee. Dr. Lipoti has served on the Food and Drug Administration's Technical Electronic Product Radiation Safety Standards Committee. She was elected to the National Council on Radiation Protection and Measurement in 2002, where she has served on the board of directors and the budget and finance committee. Currently, she is a member of the Advisory Panel on Public Policy and Scientific Committee 6-2, Radiation Exposure of the U.S. Population. Dr. Lipoti participated in the Improvised Nuclear Device Exercise conducted in New Jersey in November 2007.

John MacKinney, M.S., M.P.H., is a senior policy advisor and deputy director for nuclear and radiological policy in the Department of Homeland Security, where he coordinates interdepartmental and interagency programs and policies in radiological and nuclear terrorism prevention and response. Mr. MacKinney has 20 years of experience in radiation science and policy in areas including nuclear facility decommissioning, radiological risk assessment, standards and regulations, research and development, and nuclear/radiological homeland security science and policy. He previously worked at EPA's National Homeland Security Research Center, where he led a team of researchers investigating scientific solutions for radiological dispersal device (RDD) and IND attack response and recovery. Mr. MacKinney has served as an expert consultant to the World Bank on environmental radiological issues and on a number of senior-level White House working groups, including the Homeland Security Council (HSC) Scenarios Writing Group, the National Security Council/HSC Counterproliferation Technology Coordination Committee, the Office of Science and Technology Policy (OSTP) RDD/IND Working Group, and the OSTP Nuclear Defense Research and Development/Response and Recovery Working Group. He holds a B.S. in geology from Wheaton College (Wheaton, Illinois), an M.S. in geophysics from the University of Wisconsin, and an M.P.H. from the Johns Hopkins University School of Public Health. Mr. MacKinney is certified in risk assessment and risk policy through the Risk Sciences and Public Policy Institute. His current interests are science, technology, programs and policy for nuclear and radiological terrorism prevention, and consequences management.

Carmen T. Maher (Commander, U.S. Public Health Service), B.S.N., M.A., RN, RAC, is a senior nurse officer in the U.S. Public Health Service Commissioned Corps and currently serves as a regulatory policy analyst in the Food and Drug Administration's (FDA's) Office of Counterterrorism and Emerging Threats in the Office of the Commissioner. Commander Maher collaborates with senior agency staff in developing and updating agency and interagency counterterrorism and chemical, biological, radiological, and nuclear consequence management and mitigation policies and plans. Prior to joining FDA, Commander Maher was assigned to the National Institute of Allergy and Infectious Diseases, Division of Microbiology and Infectious Diseases, as a lead regulatory officer for pre-clinical and early clinical development of vaccines and therapeutics to prevent or treat illnesses caused by smallpox, anthrax, and influenza disease agents. As a federal first responder, Commander Maher has assisted state and local response efforts and was an active member of the PHS-1 Disaster Medical Assistance Team, serving on its leadership cadre for 2 years. Commander Maher earned her M.A. in national security and strategic studies with highest distinction from the U.S. Naval War College, Rhode Island. She earned her B.S.N. and her associate degree in life sciences from the University of Puerto Rico. She holds a Regulatory Affairs Certification in U.S. health care products regulations.

John Mercier (Colonel, U.S. Army), Ph.D., PE, DABR, is the lead DoD subject matter expert for nuclear weapons effects on humans. His current work includes mass casualty care and protective actions following an urban nuclear detonation. He currently serves at the Armed Forces Radiobiology Research Institute as institute nuclear consultant and director emeritus of the Military Medical Operations Directorate, with oversight of the Medical Effects of Ionizing Radiation Course, the Medical Radiobiology Advisory Team, and radiological safety operations for institute nuclear and radiation facilities. Previous duties have included serving as radiological consultant to the Multinational Corps-Iraq, NATO senior umpire for the Sampling and Identification of Radiological Agents, leader of the U.S. Army Radiological Advisory Medical Team, chief of Health Physics at the Walter Reed Army Medical Center, and chairman of DoD's Nuclear Weapons Effects Human Response Panel. Colonel Mercier is a licensed nuclear engineer, nuclear plant senior reactor operator, and medical physicist. He is also board certified in diagnostic radiological physics and medical nuclear physics. Colonel Mercier has nearly 30 years of military service, he holds a Bronze Star from his combat tour with the XVIII Airborne Corps, and his military retirement has been approved for 2009.

Joseph S. Newton is the recipient of the 2006 Medal of Valor for the State of Illinois and is a decorated firefighter/paramedic who works for the Chicago

Fire Department and neighboring suburb of Westmont, Illinois. His educational background includes Illinois State Paramedic, Firefighter II, Firefighter III, Hazmat Operations including Computer-Aided Management of Emergency Operations training, EMT Lead Instructor, Fire/EMS Instructor I, and Instructor II, among other various certificates and training, such as emergency response to terrorism, rescue dive, advanced cardiac life support, pediatric education for prehospital professionals, and international trauma life support. In his duties with the Chicago Fire Department, Mr. Newton is a paramedic assigned to the Operations Division, and he is currently detailed to Fire Academy South/EMS Training where, as an instructor, he has held a direct supervisory role in the training of all new fire and EMS hires for the past 4 years. He is also a field training officer responsible for District 1 Operations, consisting of approximately 1,000 department members. District 1 encompasses the downtown metropolitan area of Chicago, including 22 engine companies, 11 truck companies, 1 squad company, Air Sea Rescue, 13 ambulance companies (3 BLS, 10 ALS), Hazardous Materials Team 511, Fire Prevention Bureau, Training Division, Headquarters, Air Mask (Support Services), Special Events Response Teams, Public Education, Internal Affairs, and the Photo Unit. Mr. Newton has trained to work as a liaison for the Chicago Fire Department Tactical Operations Intelligence Center and has had hands-on experience as a member of small special operations disaster deployment teams consisting of 30 members. He has also been tasked with the management and deployment of on-scene field resources for large-scale special events, ranging from 20,000 to 1.2 million civilian participants, held inside and outside of the City of Chicago.

Ann E. Norwood (Colonel-Retired, U.S. Army), M.D., is senior associate at the University of Pittsburgh Medical Center's Center for Biosecurity in Baltimore, Maryland. She received her A.B. in psychobiology from Vassar College and her M.D. from the Uniformed Services University of the Health Sciences (USUHS), Bethesda, Maryland. Dr. Norwood completed her residency in psychiatry at Letterman Army Medical Center in San Francisco, California. She was the chief of psychiatry at Darnall Army Community Hospital, Ft. Hood, Texas, before her appointment as an assistant professor at USUHS in 1988. Dr. Norwood held a number of positions while at USUHS, including associate chair and a 6-month term as acting chair of the Department of Psychiatry. In 2003 she was assigned to Walter Reed Army Medical Center with duty at HHS as a senior advisor on risk communication to OPHEP. Dr. Norwood retired from the Army Medical Corps as a colonel and joined HHS as a civilian in 2004. Her final position in the former OPHEP (now ASPR) was as a senior policy analyst in the Office of Preparedness and Emergency Operations/Office of Preparedness Planning. Dr. Norwood is a former chair of the American Psychiatric Association's

Committee on Psychiatric Dimensions of Disaster. She is an associate editor of the peer-reviewed journal *Biosecurity and Bioterrorism: Biodefense Strategy, Practice, and Science*. She has coedited four books and published numerous articles and chapters on the behavioral health aspects of trauma associated with war, terrorism, and disasters, as well as the unique stresses associated with military service. Her other professional interests include crisis communication, resilience, and mass fatality management.

Jeanine Prud'homme is a certified industrial hygienist who serves as the assistant commissioner for the New York City (NYC) Department of Health and Mental Hygiene's Bureau of Environmental Emergency Preparedness and Response (BEEPR) and who has overseen the agency's Office of Radiological Health. With the NYC Fire Department, Ms. Prud'homme serves as the cochair of the NYC Police Department's Securing the Cities Radiological Response and Recovery Subcommittee. BEEPR's responsibilities include all hazards field and technical planning and response to environmental public health incidents. Within the Department of Health and Mental Hygiene, she plays a major role in the planning and mitigation of biological and radiological incidents in NYC.

Irwin Redlener, M.D., FAAP, is associate dean, professor of clinical public health, and director of the National Center for Disaster Preparedness at Columbia University. Dr. Redlener speaks and writes extensively on national disaster preparedness policies, pandemic influenza, the threat of terrorism in the United States, and related issues. He is also president and cofounder of the Children's Health Fund and has expertise in health care systems, crisis response, and public policy with respect to access to health care for underserved populations. Dr. Redlener, a pediatrician, has worked extensively in the Gulf region following Hurricane Katrina, where he helped establish ongoing medical and public health programs. He also organized medical response teams in the immediate aftermath of the World Trade Center attacks of 9/11 and has had disaster management leadership experience internationally and nationally. Dr. Redlener is the author of *Americans at Risk: Why We Are Not Prepared for Megadisasters and What We Can Do Now*, published in August 2006.

Dori B. Reissman (Captain, U.S. Public Health Service), M.D., M.P.H., has been providing leadership and vision to integrate health, safety, and resiliency into incident management strategies for emergency responders and address organizational dynamics affecting traumatic stress for workers in hazardous occupations. Contributions include emergency response service, expert consultation, applied behavioral research, and policy guidance. She initiated efforts to address community resiliency as a public health protection strategy as well as to address organizational and workforce resilience at CDC, and she has supported numerous public health missions in response to natural disasters and terrorist attacks. She was commissioned as a medical officer in the Public Health Service in 1997, when she joined CDC as an epidemic intelligence officer. Dr. Reissman completed residency training in occupational and environmental medicine in 1997, including an M.P.H. at the University of Illinois. Previously, she had completed residency training in psychiatry and provided psychiatric consultation services in private and faculty-based practices in addition to teaching and supervisory positions in university-affiliated hospitals. Dr. Reissman was chief of the emergency psychiatric services at St. Vincent's Hospital and Medical Center of New York when the 1993 World Trade Center bombing incident occurred. She received a medical degree from Albert Einstein College of Medicine, New York, in 1984. Prior to her medical training, Dr. Reissman obtained a B.S. in environmental sciences from Cook College, Rutgers University, in New Jersey, and an M.A. in pharmacology and toxicology from Columbia University in New York.

Alan L. Remick is the consequence management program manager for the Office of Emergency Response, National Nuclear Security Administration (NNSA). Mr. Remick has more than 25 years of technical and program management experience in emergency response. Prior to working for the Department of Energy (DOE) NNSA, he managed the nuclear emergency monitoring and assessment program at Mare Island Naval Shipyard. At DOE/NNSA, he manages the Consequence Management Program, which provides expert technical advice and assistance from the DOE/NNSA complex in response to radiological accidents, lost or stolen radioactive materials, and acts of nuclear terrorism. He received a B.S. in nuclear engineering from Kansas State University.

Adela Salame-Alfie, Ph.D., is the assistant director of the Division of Environmental Health Investigation in the New York State Department of Health (NYSDOH). Prior to that appointment she was the director of the Bureau of Environmental Radiation Protection at NYSDOH. Dr. Salame-Alfie is the current chair-elect of the Conference of Radiation Control Program Directors. She is also chair of the Homeland Security Emergency Response 2 Committee that was responsible for the preparation of the *Handbook for Responding to a Radiological Dispersal Device—The First 12 Hours.* Dr. Salame-Alfie is a member of the National Council on Radiation Protection and Measurements' (NCRP's) Scientific Committee SC4-2, "Population Monitoring and Decontamination Following a Nuclear or Radiological Incident," and is also a member of the American Society for Testing and Materials' E54.2 committee that developed the *Standard*

Practice for Radiological Emergency Response. Dr. Salame-Alfie received her M.S. and Ph.D. in nuclear engineering from Rensselaer Polytechnic Institute in Troy, New York.

Aashish Shah, M.D., J.D., FACOG, is the regional medical director for Health Service Region 6/5S in the greater Houston, TX, area. Formerly, he served as the senior policy advisor for health and medical preparedness for the Texas Department of State Health Services, where his responsibilities included the evaluation and development of health and medical prepared-ness policy for the department. In addition, he is the associate director of public health preparedness at the University of Texas School of Public Health Center for Biosecurity and Public Health Preparedness. He previ-ously served as the chief physician for public health preparedness at the City of Houston Department of Health and Human Services. As a board-certified obstetrician-gynecologist and a fellow of the American College of Obstetricians and Gynecologists, Dr. Shah has had experience in both private and public health sectors. He began his career in private practice in League City, Texas. He then worked at the University of Texas Medical Branch Women's HealthCare Group and was a clinical assistant professor. Dr. Shah completed his B.A. in biology from the University of Texas in Austin, his M.D. from the University of Texas Health Science Center in San Antonio, and his residency in obstetrics, gynecology, and infertility at the University of Texas Health Science Center Houston. He recently graduated from the University of Houston Law Center with an emphasis in health policy, where he authored *HIPAA and Hurricanes Katrina and Rita: A Primer for Disclosure of Protected Health Information to the Local Pub-lic Health Authority.* Dr. Shah has had experience working with the state legislature. As a legislative intern with the Texas Medical Association, he worked with the House Subcommittee on Public Health to establish the Council on Cardiovascular Disease and Stroke.

Katherine Uraneck, M.D., is the senior medical coordinator for the New York City Department of Health and Mental Hygiene in the Healthcare Emergency Preparedness Program. Her primary focus areas include radi-ation incident planning and response, hospital surge capacity, pediatric preparedness, and mass fatality planning. She has been project manager, coauthor, and editor of *NYC Hospital Guidelines for Responding to a Contaminating Radiation Incident* as well as an active participant in the New York City Securing the City subcommittee on the city's response to a radiation incident. Nationally Dr. Uraneck has participated in the Center for Biosecurity's Working Group on Emergency Mass Critical Care, the CDC Working Group on Radiation Population Monitoring, and the NCRP Scientific Committee 4-2, "Population Monitoring and Decontamination

Following a Nuclear or Radiological Incident." Dr. Uraneck is a board-certified and residency-trained emergency physician. She completed her undergraduate degree in biomechanical engineering at Cornell University, her M.D. at Washington University Medical School in St. Louis, Missouri, and her residency and fellowship in emergency medicine at the Medical College of Pennsylvania in Philadelphia. She practiced as an emergency physician in Philadelphia, Pennsylvania; in Albany, New York; and in rural Vermont. In 2002, Dr. Uraneck completed a master's degree in journalism at the Columbia University Graduate School of Journalism.

Reuben K. Varghese, M.D., M.P.H., promotes disease control and prevention and overall community health as chief of the Public Health Division of Arlington County, Virginia. Varghese began his career at a health maintenance organization, where he served as internist. He served as chief of the Medical Affairs and Surveillance Branch of the Food Safety and Inspection Service at the Department of Agriculture (USDA) from 2004 to 2005. From 2000 to 2002 he was an epidemic intelligence service officer for CDC. While at CDC, he was part of a team sent to New York City to monitor latent health effects caused by 9/11—an asset to a community such as Arlington, which also was directly affected on 9/11. Prior to his work at USDA, Dr. Varghese was director of the Three Rivers Health District based in Middlesex County, Virginia, from 2002 to 2004. He received his M.D. from Brown University and has an M.P.H. from the Johns Hopkins University School of Hygiene and Public Health.

Michael Welling has served as the director of the Virginia Radioactive Materials Program (RMP) for 2 years. RMP was created in order for Virginia to become an agreement state and regulate all radioactive material in the commonwealth. Prior to this, Mr. Welling worked for the Wisconsin Radioactive Materials Program for 5 years. Mr. Welling was a nuclear electrician in the U.S. Navy for 6 years. He has a B.A. in business management from Lakeland College in Wisconsin.

Albert L. Wiley, Jr. (United States Navy Reserve-Retired), M.D., Ph.D., FACR, received Board of Nuclear Engineering and postgraduate training in nuclear engineering from North Carolina State University and worked as a nuclear engineer. He later graduated from medical school at the University of Rochester, followed by an internship in surgery/medicine at the University of Virginia at Charlottesville and residency training in radiation oncology and nuclear medicine at Stanford University and the University of Wisconsin-Madison. He also received a Ph.D. (major in radiobiology, minor in nuclear engineering) at the University of Wisconsin-Madison. In the U.S. Navy, Dr. Wiley served in the United States and Europe as senior medical officer for a major Navy Radiation Accident Response Team; as medical director of the U.S. Navy Radiological Defense Laboratory, San Francisco; and as instructor at the Navy Nuclear Training Center, Naval Air Station North Island, Coronado, California. For most of his career, he was a professor of radiation oncology and human oncology at the University of Wisconsin-Madison, where he is currently emeritus professor. He is also part-time clinical professor of radiation oncology at East Carolina University. Dr. Wiley is currently the director of the Radiation Emergency Assistance Center/Training Site and the World Health Organization (WHO) Collaborating Center at Oak Ridge, as well as vice president of Radiation Emergency Medicine at Oak Ridge Associated Universities, Oak Ridge, Tennessee. He is board certified in radiation oncology (ABR), nuclear medicine (ABNM), medical physics (ABMP, medical health physics), and by ABSNM (radiation protection). He has served nationally and internationally as a consultant to the Nuclear Regulatory Commission, Department of Energy, Department of State, Department of Veterans' Affairs, HHS, WHO, and International Atomic Energy Agency.

Richard P. Zuley recently retired from the Chicago Police Department after almost 37 years of service. During the last 1.5 years of his police career, Detective Zuley was detailed to the Training Academy, where he became a state-certified instructor and served as the senior instructor and one of the developers of Chicago's highly regarded Terrorism Awareness and Response Academy. Following his retirement, Mr. Zuley was hired by the City of Chicago Department of Public Health, where he works as the senior emergency management coordinator in the Emergency Preparedness and Response Division. Mr. Zuley's duties include developing preparedness and response plans, in addition to being the primary CBRNE officer and the development of an indigenous intelligence fusion section. Earlier in his career Mr. Zuley was a Marine and still serves as an intelligence officer in the U.S. Naval Reserve. Commander Zuley has had extensive active-duty time including 2 years deployed overseas as part of Operations Enduring Freedom and Iraqi Freedom. He was closely involved in the actual intelligence collection mission and served in a leadership position in that effort. Mr. Zuley received two Defense Meritorious Service medals for his efforts in those operations. In addition to his work with the Chicago Police Department, Mr. Zuley continues to teach terrorism-related classes through the Chicago Department of Public Health, Department of Homeland Security, and multiple state agencies. He is a licensed pilot and a graduate of Dominican University with a degree in political science and history, and he also did graduate studies at National-Lewis University.

Appendix D

Biographical Sketches of Committee Members, Consultant, and Staff

COMMITTEE MEMBERS

Georges C. Benjamin, M.D. (*Chair*), became executive director of the American Public Health Association, the nation's oldest and largest organization of public health professionals, in 2002. Prior to that he was secretary of the Maryland Department of Health and Mental Hygiene, where he played a key role in developing Maryland's bioterrorism plan, following 4 years as the department's deputy secretary for public health services. Dr. Benjamin started his medical career in 1981 in Tacoma, Washington, where he managed a 72,000-patient-visit ambulatory care service as chief of the Acute Illness Clinic at the Madigan Army Medical Center. A few years later, he served as chief of emergency medicine at the Walter Reed Army Medical Center. After leaving the Army, he chaired the Department of Community Health and Ambulatory Care at the District of Columbia General Hospital. He was promoted to acting commissioner for Public Health for the District of Columbia and later directed one of the busiest ambulance services in the nation as interim director of the Emergency Ambulance Bureau of the District of Columbia Fire Department. Dr. Benjamin is a member of the Institute of Medicine (IOM) Board on Population Health and Public Health Practice. He has served on several other IOM and IOM/National Research Council committees: training physicians for public health careers; measures to enhance the effectiveness of the CDC quarantine station expansion plan for U.S. ports of entry; evaluation of the metropolitan medical response systems program; and research and development needs for improved civilian medical response to chemical or biological terrorism incidents. He also serves on the boards of Partnership for Prevention and the Regan Udall Foundation. Dr. Benjamin is a graduate of the Illinois Institute of Technology and the University of Illinois College of Medicine. He is board certified in internal medicine and is a fellow of the American College of Physicians and a fellow emeritus of the American College of Emergency Physicians. He is an IOM member.

George J. Annas, J.D., M.P.H., is the Edward R. Utley Professor and chair of the Department of Health Law, Bioethics and Human Rights, at the Boston University School of Public Health and professor at the Boston University School of Medicine and School of Law. He is the cofounder of Global Lawyers and Physicians, a nongovernmental organization dedicated to promoting health and human rights. Dr. Annas is an expert on health law, bioethics, and international human rights, is the author or editor of 17 books, including *The Rights of Patients, American Bioethics, Some Choice,* and *Standard of Care,* and writes a regular feature, "Health Law, Ethics, and Human Rights," for the *New England Journal of Medicine.* He is a fellow of the American Association for the Advancement of Science, a member of the National Academies' Committee on Human Rights, and cochair of the American Bar Association's Bioethics and Health Rights Committee (Individual Rights and Responsibilities Section). Dr. Annas holds degrees in economics (A.B.), public health (M.P.H.), and law (J.D.) from Harvard University. He is an IOM member.

Donna F. Barbisch (Major General Retired), C.R.N.A., M.P.H., D.H.A., is among the nation's most distinguished experts on terrorism, disaster preparedness, and national and international security interoperability. She is president of Global Deterrence Alternatives, LLC, and director of the Institute for Global and Regional Readiness. With more than 20 years of experience in managing complex private and public medical and organizational challenges, she addresses the complexities of combating terrorism through comprehensive planning and culture change. She provides visionary policy and program integrating solutions related to the national security threats of terrorism, natural disasters, and emerging infectious diseases. Dr. Barbisch focuses on strategic planning for reducing threats and responding to crises with multilevel and multijurisdictional elements. She develops and implements holistic management programs that promote interoperability across civilian and military organizations as well as political and business environments that result in strategic partnerships. Major General Barbisch served in a multitude of active and reserve military assignments, from Vietnam to the Pentagon. Her final military assignment was as director of Chemical, Biological, Radiological, and Nuclear Program Integration for the Office of the Secretary of Defense. She has a bachelors degree from

California University of Pennsylvania, an M.P.H. from the University of North Carolina at Chapel Hill, and a D.H.A. in health administration from the Medical University of South Carolina.

Frederick M. Burkle, Jr., M.D., M.P.H., D.T.M., is actively involved in research, policy issues, and writing in a number of areas, including globalization and health; globalization and disaster management; global/international health as it pertains to war, conflict, recovery and rehabilitation, refugee care, and vulnerable populations; pandemics/epidemics; primarily population-based care and triage management; civil-military cooperation and collaboration; tropical medicine and bioterrorism; United Nations reform; and the United Nations (UN)/World Health Organization (WHO)/United Nations Childrens' Fund response and international health regulations in global health crises. A retired professor from the University of Hawaii John A. Burns School of Medicine, he is currently a Woodrow Wilson International Scholar and senior fellow, Harvard Humanitarian Initiative, Harvard University, and associate scientist, Johns Hopkins University Medical Institutions. He is a retired Naval Reserve Captain and former deputy assistant administrator, Bureau of Global Health, U.S. Agency for International Development. He received his M.D. from the University of Vermont College of Medicine; his M.P.H. from the University of California, Berkeley; a diploma in health emergencies in large populations from the University of Geneva; and a diploma in tropical medicine from the Royal College of Surgeons in Dublin. He is qualified in emergency medicine, pediatric emergency medicine, pediatrics, and psychiatry. Dr. Burkle is an IOM member.

Colleen Conway-Welch, Ph.D., RN, FAAN, FACNM, has served as professor and dean of the Vanderbilt University School of Nursing since 1984. She has been active in nursing practice and nursing education for more than four decades. The holder of three honorary doctorates from Cumberland University, Georgetown University, and the University of Colorado, she is a graduate of Georgetown University, Catholic University of America, and New York University. She has published extensively, served on President Reagan's Commission on the HIV Epidemic in 1988, the National Bipartisan Commission on the Future of Medicare in 1998, and the Governor's Tennessee Commission on the Future of TennCare, and was appointed by Health and Human Services Secretary Tommy Thompson to the Secretary's Council on Public Health Preparedness, Office of the Assistant Secretary for Public Health Emergency Preparedness. She is also a member of the Medicare Coverage Advisory Committee with the Department of Health and Human Services (HHS) and a member of the George Washington University Homeland Security Policy Institute. She was named by President Bush and confirmed by the U.S. Senate in

2006 as a member of the Board of Regents of the Uniformed Services University of the Health Sciences. In 2007, she was appointed by Secretary Leavitt of HHS to the Advisory Committee to the Director of the National Institutes of Health (NIH). She is a former president, and one of the founders, of Friends of the National Institutes of Health, National Institute for Nursing Research. She is an invited member of the Governor's Office of Children's Care Coordination and member of the Board of Commissioners of the Tennessee Safety Seismic Commission panel of advisors. She is a fellow in the American Academy of Nursing, a charter fellow of the American College of Nurse-Midwives, and serves as a director on the boards of Pinnacle Bank, RehabCare Group, and Ardent Health Services, in addition to numerous other 501(c)3 boards, such as the Health Care Leadership Council in Washington, DC. She is also the founding director of the Nursing Emergency Preparedness Education Coalition. Dr. Conway-Welch is an IOM member.

Daniel F. Flynn, M.D., is a board-certified radiation oncology physician on staff at Caritas Holy Family Hospital and Medical Center in Methuen, Massachusetts. He is an active lecturer on the visiting faculty at the Radiation Assistance Center and Training Site in Oak Ridge, Tennessee. He serves as the medical consultant to the state of Massachusetts on its nuclear incident advisory team. As a colonel in the U.S. Army Reserves Medical Corps, he has been an invited contributor to the armed services training manuals on the subject of the medical management of mass casualties from a nuclear event, and he has been an invited lecturer at the Armed Forces Radiobiological Research Institute. He also has been both triage officer and deputy commander of a combat support hospital and is a 2007 Iraq War veteran. Dr. Flynn received his M.S. in medical radiation physics from the Harvard School of Public Health and his M.D. from Jefferson Medical College, and he did postgraduate training at Massachusetts General Hospital, where he later served on the staff with an academic appointment to Harvard Medical School.

Richard J. Hatchett, M.D., joined the Office of the Director at the National Institute of Allergy and Infectious Diseases (NIAID) in July 2005, where he became associate director for Radiation Countermeasures Research and Emergency Preparedness in the Division of Allergy, Immunology, and Transplantation. In late 2005 and early 2006 he served on the White House Homeland Security Council as Director for Biodefense Policy. Prior to joining NIAID, he served as senior medical adviser in the HHS Office of Public Health Emergency Preparedness. He received his medical degree from Vanderbilt University and completed postgraduate training in internal medicine at Weill Cornell Medical Center in New York and in medical oncology at the Duke University Medical Center.

Fred A. Mettler, Jr., M.D., is chief of radiology and nuclear medicine at the New Mexico VA Health Care System and is a professor at the University of New Mexico Health Sciences Center in Albuquerque. His area of expertise is the medical effects of ionizing radiation. He is the U.S. representative to the UN Scientific Committee on the Effects of Atomic Radiation, an emeritus commissioner of the International Commission on Radiological Protection, and a member of the National Council on Radiation Protection and Measurements. Dr. Mettler has served as a consultant to WHO and the International Atomic Energy Agency. He was the Health Effects Team Leader for the International Chernobyl Project and is an academician of the Russian Academy of Medical Sciences.

Judith A. Monroe, M.D., was appointed in March 2005 by Governor Mitch Daniels as the Indiana State Health Commissioner and medical director of Medicaid. She is president of the Association of State and Territorial Health Officials (ASTHO) and served as the chair of the ASTHO Preparedness Policy Committee. During her tenure as health commissioner she has played a key role in improving public health preparedness in Indiana, and in December 2006 she traveled to Israel with a delegation from ASTHO for preparedness training. She is chair of the executive board of the Indiana Tobacco Prevention and Cessation Agency and is a member of the Public Health Accreditation Board and the Indiana Health Information Exchange. Dr. Monroe is a family physician and National Health Service Corps scholar. She started her career in 1986 providing health care in rural Appalachia, during which time she was featured with former Surgeon General C. Everett Koop in a documentary on the heath care crisis in America. In 1990 she joined the faculty of the Indiana University School of Medicine and served as clinical director with the Department of Family Medicine. In 1992 she joined the medical staff of St. Vincent Hospital in Indianapolis and became the director of the Family Medicine Residency Program and Primary Care Center. In this role she oversaw multidisciplinary ambulatory services with more than 50,000 visits per year. Dr. Monroe received her undergraduate degree from Eastern Kentucky University and is a graduate of the University of Maryland School of Medicine. She did her postgraduate training at the University of Cincinnati and is a fellow of the American Academy of Family Practice.

Paul E. Pepe, M.D., M.P.H., oversees one of the nation's largest academic emergency departments (55 faculty, 70 residents and fellows) at the extremely busy county (public) emergency-trauma center (Parkland Hospital) and the North Texas Poison Control Center. He is also the director of medical emergency services for public safety, public health, and homeland security in the Office of the City Manager for the City of Dallas and the jurisdictional medical director for the regional BioTel System (a centralized emergency medical services program that includes more than 3,000 firefighters, emergency medical technicians, and paramedics from the fire departments for the City of Dallas and 16 surrounding cities). He also provides medical direction for the Dallas Police Department and the Dallas Metropolitan Medical Response System for counterterrorism. In addition to a distinguished, productive career in academic medicine (with nearly 500 published scientific papers and abstracts including multiple landmark publications in multiple disciplines), Dr. Pepe has simultaneously served as a high-level municipal or state employee for a quarter century, managing large public budgets but doing so in an in-the-trenches, "street-wise" manner. He is renowned for a grassroots approach to planning, implementing, and overseeing a systems approach to saving lives, both operationally and through clinical trials. His programs have resulted in some of the highest reported cardiac-arrest and trauma survival rates among all large U.S. metropolitan cities. He was a senior author on the original American Heart Association *Chain of Survival* publication (1991), a reference now cited symbolically in nearly every CPR-related publication and training course worldwide, and he has served for many years as emergency medicine and trauma consultant for the U.S. Secret Service, the White House Medical Unit, the National Institutes of Health, and network news organizations.

Thomas M. Seed, Ph.D., is currently a consultant in the general area of radiation medical countermeasures, having retired at the end of 2007 as the associate director of research of the Radiation Effects Research Foundation (RERF) in Hiroshima, Japan. Prior to the RERF appointment, he held the following professional appointments: research professor/senior scientist, Radiation Biophysics/Vitreous State Laboratory, Catholic University of America, Washington, DC (2003-2005); group leader/senior scientist, radiation medical countermeasures, Armed Forces Radiobiology Research Institute, Bethesda, Maryland (1996-2003); research scientist/group leader, radiation hematology, Division of Biological and Medical Research, Argonne National Laboratory, Argonne, Illinois (1975-1995); and assistant scientist/ department chairman, biological ultrastructure, Blood Research Laboratory, National Red Cross, Bethesda, Maryland (1973-1975). He currently serves as a council member of the National Council on Radiological Protection and Measurements as well as a member of the Stem Cell Radiobiology Working Party of the International Commission of Radiological Protection, and previously he served on the North Atlantic Treaty Organization-related research study groups that focused on radiation injury and medical countermeasures. In addition to his research interest in the nature and mechanisms of action of radioprotective agents, he also has an interest in structural and function studies of radiation-induced hematopathology, cellular mechanisms of pre-clinical phase leukemogenic processes, and mechanistic studies on red cell destruction during infectious hemolytic anemias. Dr. Seed earned his B.A. from the University of Connecticut and his M.S. and Ph.D. (microbiology) from Ohio State University.

James M. Tien, Ph.D., E.E., S.M., B.E.E., became dean of the University of Miami College of Engineering in September 2007. An internationally renowned researcher, he formerly served as the Yamada Corporation Professor at Rensselaer Polytechnic Institute and was founding chair of its Department of Decision Sciences and Engineering Systems and professor in its Department of Electrical, Computer, and Systems Engineering. Dr. Tien joined the Rensselaer faculty in 1977 and twice served as its acting dean of engineering. In 2001 he was elected to membership in the National Academy of Engineering, one of the highest honors accorded to an engineer. His research interests include systems modeling, public policy, decision analysis, and information systems. He has served on the Institute of Electrical and Electronics Engineers Board of Directors (2000-2004) and was its vice president in charge of the Publication Services and Products Board and the Educational Activities Board. Tien earned his bachelor's degree in electrical engineering from Rensselaer and his Ph.D. in systems engineering and operations research from the Massachusetts Institute of Technology.

Robert J. Ursano, M.D., is professor of psychiatry and neuroscience and chairman of the Department of Psychiatry at the Uniformed Services University of the Health Sciences in Bethesda, Maryland. He is also director of the Center for the Study of Traumatic Stress. He has served as the Department of Defense representative to the National Advisory Mental Health Council of the National Institute of Mental Health (NIMH) and is a past member of the NIMH Rapid Trauma and Disaster Grant Review Section. Dr. Ursano is the editor of the journal *Psychiatry* and senior editor of the *Textbook of Disaster Psychiatry*. He has received the Department of Defense Humanitarian Service Award and a Lifetime Achievement Award from the International Society for Traumatic Stress Studies. Dr. Ursano is widely published in the field of posttraumatic stress disorder (PTSD) and the psychological effects of terrorism, bioterrorism, traumatic events and disasters, and combat. He has been a member of many national advisory boards related to mental health including the IOM Committee on Psychological Responses to Terrorism and the Committee on PTSD and Compensation. He was a physician in the U.S. Air Force, retiring after 20 years service with the rank of colonel. Dr. Ursano received his M.D. from Yale University.

CONSULTANT

William F. Stephens has managed the advanced practice center at Tarrant County Public Health, working in the area of public health preparedness and new product development, for nearly 5 years. Tarrant County Public Health is one of eight centers nationwide funded by the Centers for Disease Control and Prevention and the National Association of County and City Health Officials to enhance public health preparedness through innovation. His areas of focus have been in chemical/radiological training and exercises as well as biosurveillance system development and evaluation. Prior to joining Tarrant County Public Health, Mr. Stephens worked in senior management roles in the scientific/biomedical imaging industry and in several defense systems programs. He contributed to product development for the first commercially available digital mammography systems and for image sensors used in the Human Genome Program. He holds an M.S. degree from Texas Tech University, Lubbock.

STAFF

Michael McGeary is a senior program officer at the Board on Health Sciences Policy and director of the nuclear detonation committee. He is a political scientist specializing in science, health, and technology policy analysis and program evaluation. Before 2004 he was an independent consultant for 9 years to government agencies, foundations, and nonprofit organizations in issues of science and technology. Between 1981 and 1995 Mr. McGeary was at IOM and the National Academy of Sciences, where he was staff director of more than a dozen major reports on such topics as federal funding of research and development; graduate education and employment of scientists and engineers; and priority setting, funding, and management of the National Institutes of Health. From 2004 to 2007 he was staff director for IOM committees that recommended improvements in the systems for determining disability at the Social Security Administration and the Department of Veterans Affairs. Mr. McGeary is a graduate of Harvard University and has completed all requirements for a doctorate in political science from Massachusetts Institute of Technology except the dissertation.

Susan R. McCutchen is a senior program associate at the Board on Health Sciences Policy. She has been on staff at the National Academies for 28 years and has worked in several institutional divisions and with many different boards, committees, and panels within those units. The studies in which she has participated have addressed a broad range of subjects and focused on a variety of issues related to science and technology for international development, technology transfer, aeronautics and the U.S. space program, natural disaster mitigation, U.S. education policy and science curricula, needle exchange for the prevention of HIV transmission, the scientific merit of the polygraph, human factors engineering, research ethics, disability compensation programs, health hazard evaluation, and medical and public health preparedness for catastrophic events. She has assisted in the production of more than 50 publications. Ms. McCutchen has a B.A. in French, with minors in Italian and Spanish, from Ohio's Miami University, and an M.A. in French, with a minor in English, from Kent State University.

Andrew Pope, Ph.D., is director of IOM's Board on Health Sciences Policy. He has a Ph.D. in physiology and biochemistry from the University of Maryland and has been a member of the National Academies staff since 1982 and the IOM staff since 1989. His primary interests are science policy, biomedical ethics, and environmental and occupational influences on human health. During his tenure at the National Academies, Dr. Pope has directed numerous studies on topics that range from injury control, disability prevention, and biologic markers to the protection of human subjects of research, NIH priority-setting processes, organ procurement and transplantation policy, and the role of science and technology in countering terrorism. Dr. Pope is the recipient of IOM's Cecil Award and the National Academy of Sciences President's Special Achievement Award.